Potholes

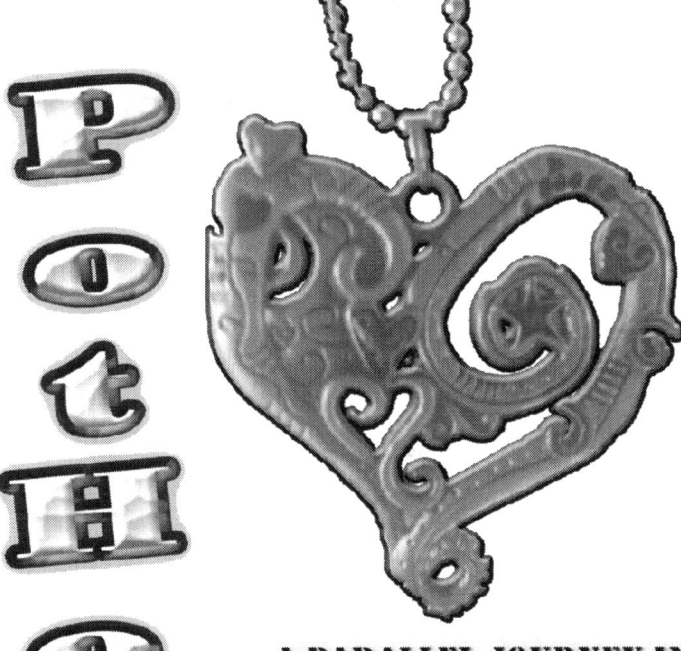

A PARALLEL JOURNEY INTO LIFE'S TRIALS, TRIBULATIONS, AND TRIUMPHS OF THE HEART.

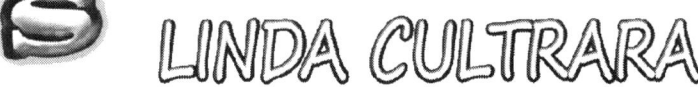

LINDA CULTRARA

POTHOLES –

a parallel journey into life's trials, tribulations, and triumphs of the heart.

Copyright © 2012 by Linda Cultrara

All rights reserved. No part of this book may be used or reproduced, in any manner whatsoever without written permission except in the case of brief quotations embodied in critical articles and reviews

Printed in the USA

Library of Congress Control Number: 2012934710

ISBN: 978-1470191962

Dedication

I dedicate my story to the memory of my cousin Sharon who passed away on September 10, 2009. She was the "pioneer" in our family, the first to receive a transplant and her journey inspired so many people to live their lives to the absolute fullest. Each moment of the 29 years she lived post transplant was a blessing and a path for me to follow. I may never be able to fill her shoes, but I am a better person by having had her in my life.

As I became ill, Sharon offered unconditional love, support, and empathy that helped to comfort me. She did this despite her own medical complications. After my transplant I called Sharon a few times, but we never connected. I was afforded the opportunity to see her one last time the day after she was admitted to Hospice. She died that evening in her sleep, just four months after my surgery. I felt such peace in her passing...as if she was "passing the torch." Through her, I hope to do great things.

Blessings,

Linda

Contents

Preface 1

Acknowledgements 3

1 Divined Destiny: Ailing Hearts 5

    1b And So it Begins 9

2 Believe in the Balance of a Vital Heart 33

    2b Prolonging the inevitable 39

3 A Recovering Agonal Heart 53

    3b Home is Where the Heart is 71

4 Barely Beating 83

    4b Making the Best of it 92

5 A Mending Heart 101

    5b Ease of Mind & Heart 114

6 Searching for Love on My Own 129

    6b A Self Preserving Heart 140

7 A Cold Heart: Numb to Emotion 153

    7b Beating in Vain 181

8 The Deceptive Heart 195

    8b Bypassing the Heart: Vein Stripping 216

9 The Unexpecting Heart Beats Normally 225

    9b A Heart in Trouble Letting Go 242

10 Roo's Broken Heart – When a Policy is Bad Practice ..249

    10b A Heart's New Life Flutter Within 267

11 The Connected and Forgotten Hearts 273

    11b A Heart Reborn ....…..285

12 A Fight to The End 299

    12b The Heart Fallen Victim to Rejection 308

13 Beating to A Different Beat 325

    13b A Triumphant Heart, Racing to the Finish Line..338

14 A Second Chance at Life ....…357

    14b When All is Said and Done ....…..369

Preface

Through the miracle of modern science, I am fortunate in my lifetime to be the first generation in my family to be genetically identified as having a "phospholamban" mutation affecting my heart. I think I was lucky, but others may prefer not to know.

It's fairly complicated but the rare mutation has succeeded in killing over 67% of my family at least, until 1979. The disorder impacts the way the heart utilizes calcium, or in our case traps it... Calcium normally rushes into the cardiac cell causing it to contract, and then reverses its path allowing it to rest. In my case the calcium gets stuck and the heart doesn't relax–ever. That clenched heart in turn fills in a contracted state instead of while it is relaxed. Over time the muscle becomes stretched and weak like an old balloon. Function is lost parallel to my family: dysfunction.

As exciting as it was to be included in medical journals such as Science Magazine in 2003, I knew two things about this "heart disease," as it was known in my family: I had it, and I would need a heart transplant. That was exciting to know, I think.

Before the gene was identified, life and family events were like Russian roulette, no one knew who was next and who would be absent at the next celebration. Our accepted norm was, "Here today gone tomorrow."

Congestive heart failure, cardiomyopathy, and fatal arrhythmias lurked all around me. Despite knowing I had inherited the gene I made every effort to beat it. Yet destiny prevailed. In 2008 I discovered my heart was broken, but in reality it had shattered a very long time ago.

Potholes is a parallel journey into my life and the physical and emotional heartbreaks that enabled me to become the person I am today. It exposes my family, friends, and me openly in order to help others. Every attempt has been made to protect our integrity including name changes where necessary. As you read, may your life be enriched through mine? I would never wish my experience on any other person; I wouldn't trade my life for anything.

Acknowledgements:

Without my pillars of strength: My Faith, Family, and Friends, this book would not have been possible. I am especially thankful for my dear friend Eileen Needham whose vision and belief in me thrust me forward into putting my story in writing. I open my life, my pain, and my vulnerabilities to hopefully inspire others. Her insight and gifted ability to choose the right words helped bring this story to fruition.

Through this journey I was brought to my knees and forced to realize that everything I have worked for in my life could have been gone in an instant, what I thought I had figured out was a façade, and the path I thought I so carefully planned for my future was not in my control. My life has taken on a new direction and thanks to the miracle of transplant surgery, the generosity of a donor family, and the dedicated staff who saw me through the roughest journey of my life; I learned why I was meant to be here today.

Chapter 1

Divined Destiny: Ailing Hearts

The heart is the vitality of life. From the moment it begins beating in-utero, it works tirelessly nurturing the mind, body, spirit, and soul. If it ceases to function, we in turn perish. When the heart is not healthy either physically or emotionally, thriving is difficult, if not impossible. An ailing heart learns to compensate for its inadequacies or sacrifice other functions in order to survive.

In life we can learn to thrive despite not being born with the most opportune or healthy circumstances. A healthy life may not be a choice, but a happy one is.

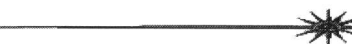

Death was in my life before I was ever born. It ran through my veins, literally and figuratively. My mother was a fraternal twin. You would think that there would be security in that simple, pure love afforded by the comfort of one another, or at least basic security. In my grandmother's womb, two lives were created, each forever entwined. Their mere existence was a divined destiny that at the time, lacked knowledge and unknowingly nurtured destruction.

Before they were born, my mom Mary and Aunt Rita grew together protected by natural law, trust and grace. Their heart beats grew in harmony, unaware of the toll their presence had taken on my grandmother's life; ignorant that she would perish when they were just three months old. With their birth, a legacy of destruction continued from an unexamined life.

Perhaps it was the physician's fault that the death certificate read, "pneumonia" and was accepted as the truth. A young mother dies leaving her infant babies and family mourning, void of her love; the very emotion they were created from. Maybe, it was because of the point that medicine was at in 1942, or just lack of medical history. It does not really matter. It happened. The events that led to her death laid the unstable foundation that later led to mine.

Then despair hovered like an ominous storm cloud, grumbling with thunderous anger, and bursting with jagged lightning bolts, repeatedly opening any healed wounds. Abuse comes in many different forms and lasts for generations. Whether created by anger, devastation, or guilt it has the power to take you as a victim, without your permission.

Turbulence and negativity bred in the early years of my mother's and her sister's lives. They were the youngest of the four children and as misfortune would have it, were perceived to be responsible for the death of their mother. It was never spoken, but everyone felt they knew the truth. They had caused her demise. This false sentiment resonated throughout the family seeping into its roots, causing instability and destruction. It carved its way throughout the family and deeply into everyone's life. Acceptance became the mechanism to massage their aching hearts while hoping to endure as a family

My grandfather, Joseph, was devastated by the loss of his beautiful wife also named Rita. Their dreams to raise a family and endure life's challenges together perished. He was left with his overwhelming responsibility of four young children, two of which were helpless infants lacking any of life's tools other than raw instinct. Joseph replaced his fond memories of her with anger; drowning his pain with alcohol. Buried with my Grandmother was his ability to love; he unknowingly allowed the pillars for his family to become emptiness, fear, and undeveloped emotional connections. In this atmosphere, nurturing was longed for, yet not found at any age, and his children grew up cultivating instability for future generations to come. It was the template for dysfunction, neglect, and abuse that prefaced my becoming an orphan; a ward of the court in my own generation.

Reflection:

I can't imagine a world in which something like my grandmother's death occurred without explanation, forewarning, understanding, or treatment options. I often wonder how she felt about her life while she was living or if she thought that she could have made a profound impact on the world. Was she content with her life being a wife and a mother? Did she lead her life determined to accomplish her dreams? Was she at least blessed with the opportunity to experience the mere joy of having her babies, or was she too weak? Did she know she was going to die and if so was she given a beautiful opportunity to appreciate each of life's moments?

My grandmother's death left no inquiry or investigation; after all it was accepted as commonplace, at the time, when people passed unexpectedly. It would not be until thirty years later when more unexplained illnesses began to rise to the surface. I wonder if things had been different, had she known her genetic template, would her choices have changed resulting in a more favorable outcome rather than a history that tells my story. Would she have chosen not to have children at all knowing the truth; would she die either way?

If life were different, maybe I wouldn't exist as I do today to write this book or reflect on what an incredible world we live in despite the things we perceive as traumatic. I wish every child were born into an opportunity that would also allow them to experience a balanced, healthy, loving life; as I had wished for my mother. If I knew how to take away her pain, loss, and emptiness and replace it with unconditional love, I would. If only she were here today maybe I could hold her and be held by her knowing what could have–should have been. Yet my story is about a much different life; my dreams, my faith and what I believe that God meant it to be.

How fortunate I am to live in a world in which in my lifetime, a genetic blueprint studied, a gene identified, carriers pinpointed, and treatment opportunities from research is available. No, it is not a perfect world, but it offers a potential treatment or cure to a family whose future generations remain fearful. In my life, the loss of life was costly, but the strides in technology…priceless.

"When the heart grieves over what it has lost, the spirit rejoices over what it has left."

-Sufi proverb

And So It Begins:

The heart functions independently through a series of involuntary chemical reactions and nerve impulses from the brain. Although there are stimuli, both internal and external in our environment that may affect the way in which it responds, we do not have the ability to control it. Very much like our lives we function as individuals with no control over what occurs, we only have the ability to control how we respond to it I have heard this expression from many people and always accepted it at face value as great words of wisdom. It wasn't until recently that I was able to fully understand how profound it really is!

For many years, I convinced myself–promised myself that if I did everything right; was a good person, a loving mother, a dedicated wife, and took care of myself, the past would not haunt me. Then there are the times like today when I realize that I never truly had any control over this promise. For me, destiny's path was too deeply etched into my foundation, and vividly imprinted within my heart.

Desperately, I was trying to go on yet would be halted in my tracks living a life that had come full circle. I had a second chance at love. I was newly re-married, working together to establish a new home with my unbelievably dashing husband, Chris. To me he was my prince charming, and my fairytale had just begun. It was 2007 and we were inseparable. At 43-years-old I thought I had finally gotten it right. In this new love, our thoughts flowed in synchronicity, no words needed to be spoken. Our relationship flourished and we worked tirelessly in our back yard, creating beauty, cultivating plants, living in harmony with nature. As I admired our accomplishments and began to reflect on how complete it all seemed, the things I loved the most resonated around me. My dogs basked in the sunshine, sprawled out on the hill behind our home just breathing in life. It seemed they had not a worry in the world and were unconditionally dedicated and peaceful. The sun shone brilliantly kissing my cheeks with its warmth. Clouds dotted the blue skies and the smell of fresh cut grass tickled my nose in the breeze. I loved the way the flowers swayed in the breeze and how their vibrant color pierced the horizon. Our home was a culmination of our cherished possessions, tastefully decorated with a spattering of our individual tastes. We melded as a couple when it came to our surroundings, enjoying traditional comfort inside and lush foliage outside. Blessed with new love our pasts were forgiven, simply being the past.

    My thoughts were interrupted as I heard the hum of the riding mower power down in front of me. Chris approached.

    "Beverage," he asked? As he spoke I inhaled the sound of his smooth, comforting voice and looked into his playful green eyes, now connecting with mine. I watched the corners of his mouth curl upward.

    He's so attentive and I am so blessed to be so in love, I thought. "Yes," I replied.

    He kissed me and headed into the house pausing only to turn back to wink at me. Mesmerized by him, I watched him struggle awkwardly up the hill missing the grace he used to have when he walked. Yet still I loved everything about him, including the way he walked, even now.

We were alone for the weekend; I called them "honeymoon days," when his boys were spending time at their mom's. Those days were cherished and carefree.

My children from my first marriage were grown, healthy, and leading independent lives of their own. This to me was a true marker of successful parenting and created less complexity in our newly blended family. Chris and I were raising his boys, now mine, which had blessed us with the opportunity to grow as a family and share a common purpose. For me, it was a new beginning.

Among these wonderful moments where everything seemed to be working smoothly the pieces of my life gently slid into place. Every day I was reminded to be thankful simply to be alive; aware of how precious each moment was, knowing my heart would someday let me know its limits.

On Memorial Day weekend, 2008, Chris and I were working together in our yard digging our pond. I was thankful that God kept him in my life. He was recovering from a snowmobile accident he had the previous winter, just five months after our wedding. In it, he shattered his femur in twelve places, broke five ribs, and bruised his kidney; injuries that I knew could've abruptly halted our lives together.

Stepping back in my memory, I began reliving that horrific day vividly recalling the day he was thrown from his snowmobile.

It was a frigid, blustery January day in Colden, New York. The wind had kicked up and the snow swirled hurriedly across the open fields limiting visibility. Chris had just purchased his new sled and it was his inaugural ride. We had on our new modular helmets so that we could communicate to one another along the ride. I loved the sport and was excited that my new "honey," as I called him, wanted to learn too. My life seemed complete. Behind him I felt empowered and protected as he led the way. I thought, *He's amazing, doing this with me and wanting to entwine my interests into his. I am blessed to have this second chance at love.* I began to concentrate more closely on the vanishing trail that the wind was now concealing, and I was no longer able to see his tail light. The reception in the headset became ear piercing and garbled. Caught now off guard, my sled had been thrown by a ditch and I prayed, "Dear God help me land this thing O.K." Elated that I was able to catch my balance after being thrust forward into the windshield with my hands clenching the handle bars, I smiled triumphantly, "Yes! I did it!"

Looking up, however I sensed something wrong. I cautiously moved forward only to see Chris' empty sled. As I exited my sled, it was difficult to see through the plumes of snow, but I noticed something black, appearing like a plastic bag rolling around on the ground ahead and thrown by the wind like tumbleweed. The static in the microphone of my helmet was unbearable and I found myself ducking my head into my shoulders trying to protect my ears.

As my vision cleared I saw the object finally halting lifeless on the frozen terrain. Panic had not yet set in. It was then I realized what the black object was. It was Chris whose body was thrown, and the screeching in my helmet was his. It was then I could make sense of that noise: screams piercing my ears as they sounded through the helmet. I feared what could be yet couldn't allow myself to process what could be.

Feeling hesitation in my steps, I approached his limp body to join Chris' side. Some of his friends quickly rode to neighboring houses to call for help as the rest of us hovered around him trying to keep him warm amidst the bone chilling nine degree day. *Chris didn't see the ditch either,* I thought. My head spun, it seemed surreal.

Chris was alert but going into shock. Rambling, he talked nonsensically about taking his helmet off. His friend Steve knew to keep his head straight and cohesively we knew the twisted fabric on his snow pants contained a severely broken leg: if not more.

"My back!" Chris yelled.

I was secretly praying it wasn't his back.

"Chris, I said calmly, "it looks like you have at least a few broken bones."

"Don't let them cut my snowmobile pants off, I know what they do in emergency rooms! And take me to Mercy hospital," he continued between his groans of agony.

Reassuringly I responded, "We will do the best we can."

The group of us stood helpless literally frozen in the moment. Chris trembled perhaps from the cold but probably more from the pain. We watched him being transferred from the field in the bed of a pickup truck, and the screams continued. This was the only way the rescue team had been able to get to us in the field.

After what seemed to be forever, we were finally on our way in the ambulance. I requested the hospital Chris wanted and the driver dropped his head.

"Ma'am," he said, "with this type of injury we will be going to the trauma center. That is Erie County Medical center (ECMC)."

"AWWWWW!" I heard his yells as the crew tried to remove his boot. The screams continued the entire ride with every movement of the vehicle...every bump in the road: screams. It unnerved and scared me.

Helplessly I watched fearing the worst as it tore at my heart. I couldn't focus on the snowmobiles we left behind or the fact that I would be alone in the hospital. I just prayed for our lives together and thanked God for his wonderful friends.

In the E.R. I sat in the waiting room trying to pull myself together. I wandered like a homeless person with our two helmets, snow pants, jackets, and his boots in hand. I held them as a child holds a teddy bear, as if they would bring me comfort.

The first physician came out telling me what she believed to be his injuries.

"He broke the hell out of his leg, and his femur is shattered. With that type of injury, we'll need to do a further work up to evaluate the damage."

A few broken ribs, a bruised kidney, and bruises the entire length of his body were a blessing compared to what could've been and I was grateful for that.

"You may go see him now, but he's pretty sedated and the orthopedic surgeon will be here soon. The femur is fractured in twelve places and the fragments will need to be aligned. He was lucky."

I saw him briefly before they took him to surgery, he was incoherent; I kissed him before they shuffled him away.

Tears now streaming down my face, I pleaded with God to allow us a future.

Once Chris was in surgery, I realized I was alone. I had no purse to call Chris's family, no support system, no car. I couldn't find the words to tell Chris' sister what had happened and how severe it was. I was just too numb. It was Chris' dad Vince who came to the hospital. Although I knew he was there for his son, I was comforted by his presence. Guilt overshadowed me, being the reason Chris was on the snowmobile in the first place. I saw Vince's anguish waiting to hear about his youngest son. The night was long and recovery would take weeks. The bruises and scars were; remnants of that infamous day.

I would complain and say that the accident caused our first year's "honeymoon" period to be cut a bit short, but after the crash he survived; I am eternally grateful he is alive today.

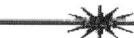

My thoughts were interrupted abruptly and I was startled back to the present hearing Chris' voice call my name. I snapped back from that formidable memory, returning to the security in the sanctuary of my yard. Looking up, our eyes again met and he reached for my hand. In his kindly eyes I saw my future and I loved what I saw.

We continued working together, Chris now helping me cultivate the soil from the pond bed we were building. He supported his weight on the tiller, somewhat symbolic of our relationship. His leg was still healing, he was in obvious discomfort now completing tasks which used to be ordinary:

now monumental. Despite his discomfort he seemed to truly enjoy my company as much I enjoyed his.

I was healthy and strong; able to complement him by shoveling dirt into the wheelbarrow and carting it into the back yard. We were having a wonderful time laughing about how some day we could look back and marvel at all the hard work we had put into it our pond, impressed by the fact we had dug it ourselves. We envisioned the babbling waterfall illuminated at night, the colorful koi swimming gracefully, and the thrill we would feel seeing frogs leaping around the periphery.

I loved Chris' outlook on life, how much he appreciated life's simple pleasures, and looked forward to our future together.

"We have a good life" he said. It's full of simple pleasures."

Inside I just knew how right he was. On so many levels, he balanced me. I just smiled and told him,

"Keep digging!"

"You have a sense of urgency like no other," he said. And I knew he was right. Unlike Chris who is well-thought and methodical. I want everything "right now" and when a thought came to mind I wanted it to come to fruition.

I now recognize that the urgency was a coping mechanism I had developed, reinforced by tragedy and loss in my life. I guess I was afraid that someday I may die not having accomplished those things I cherished and wanted to do. Chris' accident only further reinforced my fear. With his personality I found I was slowly learning to let go.

Again reminiscing, I remembered once scrambling to prepare for a family gathering. I was in a frenzy planning every intricate detail and needed to get some boxes out of storage. Drained of energy and covered in sweat, I proceeded to the basement. It was at that very moment I felt Chris' hand reach out toward me.

"Sit with me," he said.

I felt myself begin to tug away thinking, *Are you crazy?* Despite my thought, the warmth of his hand and the sincerity in his eyes had a way of helping me put my life into perspective. In his embracing arms I'd be enveloped in love beyond comprehension. We were polar opposites, but I loved the affect he had on me. All my life I clawed for this type of attention, unconditional love, and acceptance, but I didn't know how to receive it and it sometimes confused me. I loved that he held my hand every time we were together and never missed a beat to open a door. I loved that he never missed a kiss goodnight or a kiss good morning. I loved that when he'd sit up late at night and I was physically exhausted wanting to go to be, he'd pull out a blanket and pillow.

"Lay on the couch with me until I'm ready for bed. I don't want you to be alone."

He was everything to me. I had to learn to accept love without suspicion or guilt, learn that I deserved to be loved and that it was alright to relax and appreciate life's blessings. I didn't have to prove anything to him.

Over the next few days, the work in the pond became too much for me. Feeling exhausted, I began making a game out of how many shovels I could lift before getting tired and needing to rest. I ignored the shooting pains in my abdomen. I felt as if someone were standing on top of my diaphragm making it difficult to breathe. As each moment progressed, I started to feel the ache radiate through my torso, now refusing to dissipate unless I rested. I was angry that it was slowing me down; mentally convincing myself it would go away. *I can't stop now, the pond isn't finished,* I thought. This was another coping skill I developed. I would only allow myself brief intervals to remember a difficult experience or emotion and then force myself to move past it. I called it "a moment of wallowing in self-pity." Now I was far too busy to stop what I was doing and continued my quest to finish; reassuring myself that the pain would pass.

This pain was familiar. I had experienced it's intensity on a few other random occasions, yet it resolved on its own. It had a personality; each episode was short-lived, my abdomen became distended and I joked about it to Chris.

"Look at my pregnant belly," I said. "It sticks out past my toes!" Although Chris and I were both nurses, neither of us understood the pain, and as if we were playing a game, we tried to diagnose it.

Regardless, I wasn't giving in...at least not this time. It was angry and persisted driving me to a halt with increasing frequency. The protrusion hardened and became tender to the touch.

I found as time passed I was able to do less lifting and Chris and I joked about the pond.

"Well, if worse come to worse we can bury my body in this hole if die from digging this pond," I giggled.

"And no one would ever know," he said.

Another coping skill I developed was to laugh and create jokes when a situation became too uncomfortable to deal with; rather than appear weak. I rationalized with myself that the discomfort was my gallbladder and grew impatient with the fact that it waxed and waned preventing me from completing my goal. My impatience further led me to attempt to diagnose myself by testing it. I ate cheese, ice cream, and even buttered popcorn hoping to force a gallbladder attack. I thought, *If the gallbladder is gone, so too will be the pain.* I was disappointed when my efforts failed, and for the two of us as nurses, it should have been a clear cut clue.

By then we were at the point the hole for the pond was about ten feet long, eight feet wide and almost three feet deep. It was almost done, but we both realized finishing it entailed heavy labor that neither of us was capable of committing to. The heavy boulders from the yard needed to be methodically placed into the pond to create its shell and waterfall. It was difficult for me to accept failure: the project was too big for us to finish. I stood defeated knowing by this time lifting even one shovel full was laborious! Plagued with more symptoms I gave in to defeat and silently retreated into the house searching for explanation.

I continued to push through the pain and even forced myself to go to work the next day. Looking back on it now, this remains a reflection of another pattern I've created in my life; pushing forward despite the obstacles, forcing my feelings down, not admitting to needing help for fear of being perceived as weak. I refused to give in to this nagging inconvenience!

Fearing something ominous, however, I half-heartedly joked, "Chris, maybe I should go to the emergency room to get this checked out."

"Sure," he said, "but be prepared to be admitted for observation, after all you have a family history of cardiac problems."

I retracted the idea just as quickly as I mentioned it.

"I am not that sick!" I said.

While I was dressing for work the next morning I found that I could not button my pants over my rounded belly and my waistline hurt when I put pressure on it. I attempted to push past this new inconvenience by attempting to wear my "fat clothes." Valiantly I tried on several outfits resting in between each. I was forced to succumb to a loosely fitting dress with a tie that I allowed the skirt to drape loosely behind me.

Figuratively I had a bandage for everything believing that if I could cover it, it didn't exist. Within a few hours after arriving to work, reality became too hard for me to ignore. The weighted pain increased and the pressure intensified as if I were being pulled to the ground from my waistline, my body was an anchor! My knees felt as if they were struggling to keep from buckling. I was having difficulty walking around the office without becoming incredibly fatigued.

I walked to our over the counter medication supplies. *O.K., I have tried antacids, anti-gas items, histamine blockers, and basic pain meds, what is left?* I thought. Defeated, I stopped at Dave's, one of the pharmacist's desks.

"Dave, what could you suggest to ease this abdominal discomfort I'm having?"

I went on to explain the prior few days; my relenting pain, my swollen abdomen, my inability to sleep: another attempt to self-treat. Ultimately he suggested I follow up with the doctor.

I walked slowly back to my desk feeling weary. Within the hour I started to develop a cough which became congested. I felt extremely tired as a flu virus was starting and was frustrated that I could possibly be getting something. I recall thinking, *A summer cold? I don't have the time for this!* With my head now resting on my desk, a horrible memory crashed in front of my mind's eye.

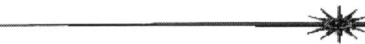

My coworker's wife had recently been hospitalized and almost died. I recalled his story through his tears, "It began with what we believed was a cold of some sort, but it resulted in a massive heart attack! She's on life support and we are not sure if she will make it." It saddened my heart to hear him break down day after day pleading with God for her recovery. I saw the devastation it caused his family.

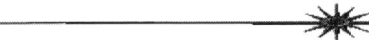

Fearing his wounds may be too fresh to be reopened watching what I was experiencing, I felt it best to remove myself from the office. Despite still denying the possibility of my symptoms being serious, out of respect for him I left to be evaluated to prevent the remote possibility of my family knowing his level of pain. I told my boss I wasn't feeling well and needed to be evaluated.

"Do you need someone to take you?" He asked.

"No thanks, I'll be fine." Even I couldn't believe what my lips were saying, yet I ventured out alone.

POTHOLES

I drove myself to an urgent care center just to ensure that I would not fall victim at work. I was afraid of being embarrassed if someone called an ambulance for me and as a result I attracted that type of attention; I couldn't bear to burden anyone with this.

The raw truth is I couldn't let my guard down for anyone. Still, as an adult, my inner child had learned to trust only myself, to take care of myself, and to lean on nobody: this ensured that no one could disappoint me and I would never again be perceived as weak.

It took three separate attempts to three medical facilities before I was fully evaluated because two of the urgent care centers were not able. The first facility was on a lunch break and would be closed for an hour. I didn't want to wait; I just wanted to be reassured that I was alright and healthy enough to return to work. The second facility was experiencing trouble with a broken x-ray machine so even though they saw me, they couldn't rule out any abdominal issues. Of course they offered to provide an ambulance transfer to the local hospital but I declined.

Part of me wanted to accept this as a clue that maybe, *just maybe*, I wasn't meant to be seen, I was overreacting, and perhaps I should just go home. Looking back, I realize that I have a pattern of dismissing clues and making choices that are avoidant of what I truly need in order to protect what I prefer to be. Going home would be consistent with that behavior.

By that time, however, I could have used an abdominal binder to hold up the weight and pressure on my belly. I was fairly short of breath, and began to waddle when I walked. "Not too much longer and this baby will be delivered," I joked to myself. Again, the attending physician asked if they could call an ambulance to transport me and I graciously declined. My belief as a nurse was that: ambulances are for people who are imminently ill, and that was not me. Besides, if I were that ill, wouldn't they have insisted?

I pursued the an emergency room, still convinced I was having a gallbladder attack, and called Chris at work to let him know where I was.

"Chris, I am going to be late from work. Can you please call your mom to get the boys off the bus?"

"Where are you?" He asked.

"I stopped at the E.R. to have my belly looked at."

Chris was at my side within a few minutes. When he arrived, he kissed me on the forehead.

"Everything will be fine, I'm here now." He reached for my hand. He remained right beside me. We waited two and a half hours to be seen before Chris called a doctor to the room.

"Why, with a patient with cardiac history have you not put oxygen on her or started an I.V line in? She is obviously short of breath!"

Without definitive answers, we continued to patiently wait in between the tests that were run. I was physically and emotionally exhausted.

Finally, the doctor came with results of some of the testing. "Your gallbladder looks fine, but your lungs are full of fluid. You are in congestive heart failure!"

Initially, I was having difficulty comprehending what he was saying, thinking he couldn't be talking to me; *He must have confused me with another patient.* To my chagrin, I was wrong and needed to be hospitalized.

Over the next few days, I was forced to realize that my heart could no longer provide for me; my vital heart was tired and the dreams I had begun to believe in with Chris were in jeopardy; unfinished. I had grown to love him deeper than anything I had ever known and recalled thanking God for this opportunity with him. Often I thought about how fortunate I was to be able to love again, and so completely. At that time, I was happy with each moment I was blessed with. Now I was feeling angry at God for allowing me to fall so hard for Chris, and once again it all became threatened. It seemed so cruel.

Intuitively, even though I knew this was the beginning of another journey, I was still too proud to be dependent and too stubborn to believe this would break my stride. In fact, the morning that I was discharged from the hospital, I couldn't get anyone at home to answer the phone and I refused to stay any longer than I had to. I thought to myself, *I feel great and I am ready to get back to my life, to living it to the fullest for however long I may have left.* I wanted to go home so desperately; I told my nurse that my husband had driven the car around front and I was meeting him downstairs I left, drove myself home and climbed into my bed where Chris lie sleeping. He was so exhausted; he never heard the phone ring when I called.

A few short weeks later, I followed up with a visit to my cardiologist, Dr. Spangenthal. I was thriving and we were both pleased with my progress. He asked me how I felt. Confused, I looked at him. "I don't know, I think I feel great, but when I look at my medical records, I recognize how ill I truly am. With that being said, I know I *should* feel awful. So, I guess I feel great based on what I understand of myself, but I am worse than the normal population."

He asked me, "Did you hear what you just said?"

I replied with a smile.

"Yes, it is confusing to me too!"

Before leaving he asked if I'd be comfortable coming back in six months. Something inside of me forced me to ponder his question for a moment. I am usually a very agreeable patient, trusting of the expert opinion, and very conscientious of how valuable office time is. In this case I felt glued to the examining table feeling my story needed to be heard. In my mind, I relived my past, flashing back into my memories of loss; looking reality in the eye.

With that in mind, I respectfully responded, "Could you refer me for a heart transplant evaluation? My sister Patti, and cousins Sharon, Eugene, and Susie (*so many loved ones*) had been placed on transplant lists within one year after their first episode with heart failure. I've looked at the history and this disease progresses quickly."

I shuddered thinking I would be the fifth transplant in this generation of my family. Suddenly I felt defeated as it seemed my efforts were all in vain. I had done everything to keep my heart in my body, and it failed. Had I failed at this too?

He looked at me somewhat puzzled. I knew he was reluctant.

"I sit here looking at you, the picture of health. You are only forty-four, an energetic, working patient. It makes no sense," he said.

It was true. I was an "Energizer Bunny." I worked out vigorously, ate healthy and was incredibly productive.

He then admitted, "This is a new frontier for me because I have only had one other transplant patient which I hadn't had a previous history with."

I was impressed with his honesty. He agreed to write the referral. I was thankful that he looked past the "physical me," listening to me as a patient, a patient with a hauntingly too familiar history.

Though I was given a choice of three possible transplant centers, I chose the Shapiro Cardiovascular Center (an affiliate of Brigham and Women's hospital) in Boston, Massachusetts without a moment's hesitation. I knew it was the farthest from my home and probably a hardship for my friends and family. I also knew that at the time the Cleveland Clinic was ranked number one in the country for heart transplants, but Brigham housed my genetic blueprint.

It was in 2003 that a research team contacted the living members of our family to initiate a dilated cardiomyopathy study. They strongly believed that our family could be a key to understanding this form of heart disease because the history was so reliably predictable. This is when I met Dr. Seideman (Cricket) and her nurse, Barbara from the genetics lab. It was their clinic that isolated the gene which caused guaranteed death for those affected in our family.

I was identified as having the gene and so were my two youngest children, Erin and Adam. The gene was there and would rear its ugly head at some point in our lives; that time was now for me. It was a dominant gene that would lay dormant; no one knowing what factors would trigger its deadly appearance.

"Do everything you can to keep your heart in your body for as long as you can," Cricket told me. "Also," she said, "keep a close eye on Erin, there are some early concerns."

That is exactly what I did.

Some would say the decision to go to Boston was selfish but I had a deeply engrained reason for my decision: my children. I hoped to give everything possible–including my heart–to their research believing one day the outcome for my future generations would improve. The decision forced me far from home, creating hardship for everyone involved. It was bittersweet but necessary.

Dr. Spangenthal referred me to Dr. Stevenson, Professor of Medicine at Harvard for my appointment. In October 2008, I was seen for a full cardiac work up. At that time, I was recovering from a blood clot that had found a home in the left ventricle of my heart. My fear of dying was coming to fruition as I recalled my mother's death being caused by a clot in her lung so many years ago.

Dr. Stevenson spent a great deal of time with me, her presence caring yet professional as she informed me of the steps we would take next. I endured a myriad of tests which ended up indicating that I indeed would be a candidate for a transplant. I was told that the transplant team would discuss my case, and then notify me of future plans. It didn't matter if I qualified by testing standards, the process was much greater than that. I felt insecure; *Once again I may not be good enough*, I thought. I was being tested, I needed to be approved by their panel, and nothing was in my control.

I was thankful I had taken care of myself all along; healthy organs would yield a better outcome. It was a new world of "what ifs?" There is no greater push to examine yourself as a person than a look at the possibility of dying. I prayed that my choices moving forward could be focused on love and gratitude.

Within two months I received the "official" acceptance letter to the transplant list, which was written very formally on Harvard letterhead. It reminded me of my college acceptance letter. To be honest, I wasn't sure if I should frame it or not. Even more humorous than that, when I showed it to my family they appeared confused asking if congratulations were in order. Life doesn't quite prepare you for the "etiquette" for this type of occasion.

The next step in my care was to be admitted to the hospital for testing. In general, I was quite impressed with how good I felt while I was there simply resting. I was also pleased to notice that for the first time in months; I didn't have the nausea, headaches, or fatigue I had for so long accepted as normal. My belly no longer hurt and I noticed how flabby it had become since the skin wasn't stretched out. I thought to myself, *I gave birth…but I guess right now sit-ups aren't an option.* To most women this would be a nightmare, but for me acceptance became the only option for now. I was quietly thankful for baggy hospital gowns to hide my new flaws.

One of the first tests I was scheduled for was an angiogram; a test that takes a unique look at the heart's vessels. For the normal population the procedure is uneventful with minimal discomfort. The doctors explained, "We will be accessing your femoral artery in your groin and threading a line into your heart to take a look. Afterward you will need to lie flat for four to six hours to prevent bleeding." I signed to consent for the seemingly uncomplicated procedure.

I have found it rare that I have the normal response in any situation, and the angiogram was no exception. I was told, "The vessels in your body are small but in general the procedure went well." The doctors had obtained all of the information that they needed and I was expected to endure the typical recovery. I was sent to recovery and began to experience excruciating pain! I began to panic, writhing uncontrollably as the pain escalated. I felt as if I would pass out. Just as my blood pressure began to drop and they tilted my bed lowering my head, Chris peeked in. I felt the room closing in on me and closed my eyes. He later told me how awful I looked. *DUH!* I thought.

The culprit was the sheath in my leg compressed a nerve causing this unbearable pain. The nurse apologized. "We need to leave the sheath in place until you stabilize."

In the interim I evaluated the pain. I thought, *This is nerve pain, the burning pain I had so frequently, as a nurse, heard my patients complain of.* It was not only burning, it was searing as if someone was branding me with a hot iron; drawing circles around my abdomen and down my back. The only thing missing was the smell of my burning flesh! I wanted to scream out loud, dissipating the seething pain with each outburst. Mentally, I couldn't bear the agony, yet knew it would only end if I could simply relax through it. I again closed my eyes taking in deep cleansing breaths, praying, knowing God would help me through. Within minutes, it was over. Somehow I made it though, unscathed.

Once all the testing was completed and the results were in I would be discharged to my home with the care of visiting nurses to monitor I.V. medication until my condition worsened enough to force me to live in the hospital while waiting for an organ. As unpredictable as my life became, it was for me a hopeful period in medical history and a fate much different than my grandmother's. This modern world of technology offered an opportunity for me to live and continue to raise my family while I waited for my heart to fail. I had no control over how disabling my journey would be, how long it may take, or even if I would survive. I did know that it was up to me to make the time I had the most valuable experience I could, and I tried.

Reflection:

I have learned that life is simply a series of events in which we develop who we are by taking each of our experiences, cultivating them and choosing what we want to take from them in order to become what we desire to be. We have the conscious ability to succeed, learn, grow, or weaken in the face of adversity. I was very fortunate to experience hardship early in my life because I believe it laid the foundation for me to become the strong individual I am today. Hardship became my mentor preparing me with much needed survival skills for the greater struggles in my life to come. In the grand scheme of things I had been cultivated for many years in preparation for my future.

I've heard it said, "God doesn't give you more than you can handle," and "There's always a bigger plan," but I found it very difficult to grasp these concepts, especially since experience seems to be the necessary tool required to fully understand.

Chris came in my life at a crucial point. He accepted me for who I was and knew that in our lifetime my heart would definitively fail. It was the one thing we could count on. In a new relationship, this would've scared many people away, yet he seemed willing to take the risk loving me so deeply. For both of us, our first few married years had more than the usual challenges. We promised one another a lifetime intertwined instead of a lifetime of parallel dreams. We grew stronger. I thank him for coming into my tumultuous life and riding the waves.

I know my destiny could have had a much different outcome, but I am forever grateful for my experiences, the ability to learn and grow into the person I have become, and the ability to share my story. In my lifetime, I will have been a success if I can help just one person through one bad experience or make one person smile.

In retrospect I don't believe my life has been all that bad. I've made decisions that have somehow worked out well and others which required me to re-evaluate. Life doesn't have a medication to make you function better, it just has lessons. For me, either I am a great learner or I have an incredibly dedicated guardian angel tugging me along. For now, he's not done with me yet!

"It's so important for people who are hurting to know that the story hasn't been finished. Things are terrible now, but there's more to the story."

-Dr. Richard Goodlin

Chapter 2

Believe in the Balance of a Vital Heart

The heart is designed in perfect balance. It's an amazing pump with right and left sides each designed with a specific function to supply its designated body systems. It is believed that the heart is an organ of divine attributes, a symbol of love and strong emotion. When we experience love, our hearts are known to flutter, and when we are afraid, our hearts may skip a beat. If it is deprived, it experiences pain and if it stops, we die.

For those of you who are fortunate, you were graced with the two key components of your heart to nurture your childhood development: a mother and father. Together, they create balance. I wasn't so lucky.

My first memories of my dad are fairly vague and sometimes I question if they are truly real or just images in my mind created through pictures or stories I've heard. He was 52-years-old when I was born and died when I was four. I don't remember much of him, which is truly sad for me. I loved his name though, Angelo.

There are a few memories having been formed at such a young age. I am uncertain what is truth, but at least there are some memories which are not lost or repressed.

Maybe it's a protective mechanism because at that age, there are some things you shouldn't have to remember.

I've heard that he used to sing "Oh Susannah" to my sisters and me. I envision us sitting in his lap radiant with the love shared between a father and his daughters. Maybe my dad played the guitar and maybe his voice was beautiful. I wish I knew, but I want to believe it was so.

I was told that he chased us with a belt when we misbehaved, and as the story continues I would hide under the kitchen table, and that he swatted the chairs with a belt, supposedly in jest. I recall peering through the aging white, painted chairs in that dimly lit kitchen. I still feel the fear of pain; being hit. In my child's mind I believed that if he can't get me, he can't hurt me.

As I grew, I realized that if he had wanted to he could've gotten me out from under there, but his point was made. I recognize now that hiding has been a coping skill I'd developed to protect myself, and it has become a self-preserving instinct ever since. As I grew older, the physical skill of hiding is no longer present, but has evolved into the ability to emotionally retreat allowing me the ability to avoid things I am unable to deal with at the time.

I often envisioned myself creating a "bubble" or protective wall around myself which dulled my senses, eased my pain, and slowed my ability to react; it placed my emotions at bay, out of reach, and preventing me from feeling them.

From pictures, I can see my dad was very Italian looking with curly dark hair like my son Adam, big brown eyes and high cheek bones. I have two pictures of him (both in black and white), one carving a turkey with my sisters and myself watching and the other in his Army uniform. He fought in World War II.

Seeing the pictures, I believe or want to believe, he shared important events (perhaps Thanksgiving) with us and we were a happy family. In the other picture he looked fairly young and was among other military men. I think he was quite handsome, but of course I am biased. He seemed happy, and I recognize his smile; the same as mine.

My mom wrote on my baby pictures, "She's the apple of his eye." referring to my dad and I sharing so many similarities. Supposedly, I look and behave a lot like him, yet I rely only on those two photos from so long ago and a few stories for validation, comfort, and reflection into those roots. I know for a fact, he was an engineer and worked for the Federal Aviation Agency based on his grave marker. I guess that makes me believe he was fairly intelligent and respectable. I've been told he believed I would be a doctor because as a child I seemed bright and compassionate. I have a few memories, but one more vivid than the others.

I was up in my room playing. We lived in a typical inner city home in Buffalo. The upstairs where my room was remained unfinished, with the typical dormers seen when a complete remodel isn't done. It wasn't really a room just a long open space and I don't even recall a bed being set up. It was there I would play, often alone, with my dolls pretending to take care of them; it seemed they were all I had. In fact, it is rare that I recollect being there with my sisters.

POTHOLES

I decided to walk downstairs. The stairwell was narrow with steep, wooden, creaky steps. I always took them slowly so no one would hear me. I remember the light being on in the kitchen. As I rounded the corner I could hear the dull hum of voices in the living room. Through the dimly lit, smoked-filled room, I could see silhouettes of people who I didn't recognize. They appeared like ghosts just sitting there in chairs and on couches around the living room. I visually searched for my mom but don't recall seeing her. The absence of her presence didn't concern me, it was the norm.

There was a buzz of conversation and none of it seemed discernable. To be honest I don't even know whose arms reached out and pulled me toward them. I vaguely remember something being said about dad not coming home again.

I was barely four-years-old and the statement meant nothing to me. My dad left everyday for work, and it always seemed as though he'd never get home. He worked long hours commuting to Rochester from Buffalo, so for a child my age he was gone a long time every day. This time, however, he would not come home late, or ever.

It was March, 1969; dad had a heart attack while driving home from work. Growing up, I wondered about the details of his death but was afraid to ask. Did he have the time to pull over or did the car just crash? Was he alone at the time of his death or was there time for his family to be there?

His death was a shock that left my mom alone, widowed at 27-years-old, with three girls under the age of nine. He was 56-years-old when he died, a well-established mature man my mom must've believed would take care of her. I can only imagine the daunting loss which may have brought her to relive the loss in her childhood. Only this time, she was the widow.

As far as my dad, I am saddened that he may have died alone at the roadside perhaps aware or maybe not that he was leaving his family behind. I can only imagine the loneliness he may have felt in the cold all alone; and how awful that could've been.

I wonder if it was like the movies where he hovered above the scene pleading for his life; or did he "see the light?" The funeral was not attended by us children, we weren't asked and we weren't included. Perhaps it was the right decision, maybe less traumatic, but for me it made it difficult to process dad's disappearance. I wasn't devastated; I just didn't understand why he didn't come back. It was more of a trust issue, one which gave birth to and reinforced the deeply embedded instability my sisters and I routinely experienced. Being alone was not new and I guess I was believed to be too young to understand.

I recognize now that his loss was a seed that led to trust and abandonment issues I had developed and carried with me later in life. Children want to believe their parents when they say they'll be back, but when they don't follow through, trust is lost. For me, learning to function on a further weakened trust system left uncertainty and a symbolic sense that half my heart had been damaged, numbing me emotionally.

Reflection:

Being so young when dad died, you'd think the impact would have been minimal. In fact, some people believed that and had me feeling the same. I had friends say to me, "You wouldn't know what it's like to lose your father because you never really had one." For many years I thought this was true. How could I miss what I didn't have?

I've learned it goes much deeper than that! All through my life I yearned for that closeness; the bond shared between a father and his daughter; the very foundation needed to develop a nurturing relationship in a mate. I may not have had it – but I missed it! I knew what a father should've been. I knew mine would never walk me down the aisle at my wedding or bounce my children on his knee. I knew I would never have the opportunity to be "Daddy's little girl."

If he were alive today, I would embrace the opportunity to look into his eyes perhaps to find there a reflection of myself. I would reach out to feel the energy in his touch and listen to the deep tone of his voice. I would ask him to sing "Oh Susannah," so I could hear it for myself. I would ask about the war and about his beliefs. I would love to know about his family, a family I never knew.

My Aunt Rita tells me that my son Adam looks a lot like my dad, which makes me very proud knowing that a part of my dad survives through my son. I only hope my son appreciates having two parents who love and encourage him, and that my daughters are able to appreciate having their dad in their lives.

I am thankful that I have been afforded the lesson to appreciate what I had then and what I have today. Through my experiences, I am able to accept what life is for now and all that it may offer in the future–not only for myself but for the good of others.

"To ease another's heartache is to forget one's own."

Abraham Lincoln

Prolonging the Inevitable:

A heart functions instinctively providing for itself as well as the body. When it is has a need it can't meet, other body systems are called upon to support it. It works optimally amidst a perfectly balanced homeostatic system. If only people functioned the same way. We go through life ensuring that our needs are met and if they aren't we seek alternate ways to accomplish them. What is unfortunate is that we get clouded in the difference between our wants and needs or even worse, we stop listening to our bodies and the world around us. We get so busy that we forget to nurture ourselves in order to be able to take care of others.

After coming home from the hospital in January of 2009, I worked for as long as I possibly could in order to maintain who I was; to remain whole and to deny my illness. I believed, "If I am as productive as always, I am not as sick as they say, and I will not be a hardship to my family. Dying isn't a possibility."

Another coping skill I had learned in my life was to bury myself in my work to avoid confronting the truth. This is part of my self-preservation mode. I knew it and I'm sure others did too. Yet, as long as I was able to do this, I felt some control of my life and in my mind my heart seemed to remain functional.

As long as I felt I was actively able to give something to someone, I felt like a worthwhile, contributing member of society, thus I was going to be alright. In this delusion my illness wasn't real, the doctor's were wrong, and I was content perceiving my life was intact. My efforts were a mere band-aid.

As my medical plan continued with follow-ups in Boston, I went on with my life as if I was invincible. It wouldn't be long before Dr. Stevenson would tell me otherwise. Just two months after being placed on the transplant list, she informed me it was time to start planning to leave work and begin resting my body for transplant. "Linda, your heart has declined quite significantly since we last saw you. At this point, you have very little wiggle room," she told me sitting on my bed. She held my hand as I processed what she had said, "Any questions?"

All I could muster up was a meek, "No."

I believe I was in denial all along or just not ready to admit I was that ill. Despite how grave it was becoming, I was so fortunate that this illness had progressed so slowly over those years that my body compensated amazingly well. It allowed me to lead the most productive life possible. In this timeframe I accomplished many of my lifetime dreams.

As Dr. Stevenson pointed out, my cardiac numbers certainly did not match my capabilities. In fact, because she didn't tell me directly that I needed to leave work, I felt I was safe: for a little longer. It wasn't until Carol, the nurse practitioner (N.P.) with the transplant team came into my room for a routine checkup, that reality hit.

We had a pleasant conversation and I began to tell her I was going to continue to work until I physically couldn't any longer. The look on her face reflected the startling truth, and then reality became crystal clear. One could say, "It hit the fan!" She looked at me very perplexed as if I didn't understand English, handed me my completed disability papers, and stated, "Linda, it's time." I was stunned into silence from that moment forward as Carol quietly left. Again I just didn't see the signs or want to, and needed a direct intervention to get me to see the truth.

It was difficult to process life: my life. I thought I felt good mentally, and on medication I felt good physically. It was a false sense of security and I just couldn't connect it as real.

Upon returning to home, I learned I had to make some emotional adjustments. I struggled with being alone at home with Chris at work and the boys at school. I felt useless and bored. Until then, I perceived a good portion of my lifeline to be my work and my colleagues. Work was where I buried my pain, denied my past, and where insecurities did not exist. There, I was effective and felt appreciated. At home in this state, I was a mom and wife, weakened and tired—unable to be what anyone needed.

Finally, I gave into my loneliness. Getting behind the wheel of my car, I drove to visit the pharmacy I worked at, just to see those reassuring faces I was so comfortable knowing. I used the excuse that I needed to fill prescriptions despite the fact we had door to door delivery from there; it was so much more than that. I thirsted for what was once normal, plagued somehow, feeling I would somehow be forgotten. (Solitude can play games with your psyche.)

My boss at the pharmacy, Paul, told me that many people had asked about me since I had returned home from the hospital, which helped comfort my anxiety. He then asked for my permission to let my customers and colleagues know how I was doing. From that point forward, there was an overwhelming influx of phone calls and e-mails from all directions, genuinely interested in how I was doing.

The timing couldn't have been more perfect for me to realize what a wonderful support system I had developed. All it took was minimal effort on my part: to let go of trying to handle it all on my own, for me to reach out to others, to allow them into my life, and accept their love and support. Once I opened that door, I found a sense of belonging.

As a registered nurse, I professionally and personally felt that my colleagues, family, and friends could learn and grow if we all shared my experiences together. Whether we would laugh or cry; sharing along the way by supporting one another would help us all get through this. I certainly didn't want to experience it alone! To keep us all connected; I developed a blog on a website called, "Care Pages." I provided daily entries which allowed me to share my monumental expedition with everyone step-by-step. The blog was a godsend as I became increasingly ill because not only did it reduce the number of e-mails that I had to address (I wrote one entry daily), I was comforted knowing my support system, my "audience" was there even though I couldn't see them. It was a daily ritual to keep in touch.

I learned so many lessons from the simple stories, words of wisdom, and even words of encouragement that people who cared about me shared with me. Some days, I just wanted to curl into a fetal position and cry, begging God to spare me. My prayers were not answered as I saw fit. They were instead answered with strength gained through the power of more prayer, more e-mails, and more random acts of kindness. Knowing I had this connection to my loved ones so far away, I found comfort in my weakest moments. My lifeline extended all the way to India and I recognized I was truly blessed! God had answered my prayers in his wisdom.

With my next hospitalization a Dobutamine trial began. They threaded an intravenous (I.V.) line through my jugular vein in my neck and slid it into my pulmonary artery. It was called a "P.A." line and was used to administer medication as well as monitor how well my heart pressures were doing. Every vital piece of recordable information was reflected onto a monitor of one type or another yet there was no monitor for measuring unnerved, displaced, or simply emotional absence.

The procedure for inserting the line involved injections of Lidocaine into my neck to alleviate pain. It's ironic that one must go through the experience of sharp, tearing pain to numb a specific area so that one doesn't feel the "real" pain.

Once numb, the vein is punctured. A popping, dull snap sound can be heard when the vessel is penetrated. It sounded and felt as if I had been snapped closed with those metal fasteners on baby clothes. A tube was then threaded through the opening in my neck into the heart and the line secured in place. It was a tolerable procedure on a good day requiring a basic analgesic to take the edge off.

I wasn't fond of the rigid tube that ended up protruding from my neck into my jaw line; a remnant of the procedure. It was awkward and limited the movement of my head and neck despite being securely taped into place and pinned to my hospital gown. It seemed barbaric and was very uncomfortable especially after the pain medication wore off. For me it was very painful because the nurse in the operating room inadvertently placed the transparent dressing at the puncture site over the top of all the cute little "short hairs" on the back of my neck. With each move I made, the hairs tugged or even broke tearing away from my skin. Simply holding my head in that awkward position caused discomfort. I was miserable with the dressing on and the longer I endured the pain, the weaker my tolerance to it became.

When it came time for the first dressing change, I was ecstatic! I so badly wanted the discomfort to end, not recognizing that those taped down hairs would now be pulled out as one painful conglomerate and with one nasty tug. Not only did I lose all of the neck hair, but some of the skin attached to it. It was excruciating but my neck was smooth as a baby's bottom! Be careful what you ask for!

For the first time in my life I realized that there was no going back and I was dependent on medical technology to sustain my life, and that my heart was no longer capable. The independence I had developed as a coping skill and the protective "bubble" I once relied on had been threatened. I was confined to a room with walking space limited to the length of tubing attached to my neck. I had to ring the nurses for assistance with daily living skills such as using the bathroom, washing, and eating. I was thrust into a situation of being mentally alert and capable but physically limited and not allowed. I associated it with my experience of caring for "stroke" patients with aphasia, being mentally capable, yet physically unable.

Simple tasks such as washing my face and changing my clothes had become a challenge requiring me to ask for help. I cried frequently wondering why I had led a life forced to develop the coping skills of independence and self-reliance that now needed to be unlearned. I questioned the purpose it all served. I had no wisdom or patience for this dependent role; yet I was certainly grateful to be alive. Psychologically I was reduced to that child of so long ago: afraid, hiding, and striking out when cornered. I had faith that God had a plan and I needed to remain patient.

I asked to see the hospital chaplain who came in very late one evening. Her name was Nancy. I was resting when she pulled her chair alongside my bed, the light in the halls behind her made it difficult to see her face. Her presence and voice were very calm, almost melodic, and reassuring.

"Pray that God gives you what you need, not what you want," she advised me. In my heart I wanted to be well and there seemed to be no other option that I was willing to consider. I needed time to process our conversation.

I confided in her, "Sometimes I get frustrated because I get so exhausted that I fall asleep during my prayers rendering me unable to ask God for help." I asked her, "If a prayer is too long, will He still listen?" I was feeling guilty I was asking for too much and that even in prayer I felt I was ineffective.

She replied, "How wonderful for you that you are so peaceful when you pray, that you are able to fall asleep." That simple statement was the beginning of my ability to let go and let God. It was profound beyond measure and I went to sleep that night content with myself, and comfortable with God. It was one of the first steps in my healing.

The first night on the medication I really did not feel any different, but my cardiac output (C.O.) showed a slight improvement. I told the nurse, "I can actually feel the presence of my heart beating." It was like going for the first ultrasound when expecting a baby. To be honest, it was exciting to feel it so vibrant and strong.

I was doing beautifully on the medication so the nurses began the discharge process. It seemed I had a new lease on life and God was answering my prayers. I was going home! At least I thought.

It was no surprise to myself, my friends, and family that I would have a glitch in the plan. I joked on my blog, "I went the extra mile."

When the nurses titrated, or bumped the medication dose upward, I began to feel a pulsation in my abdomen reminding me of when I was a child doing acrobatics. I would lay on my belly doing a "bunny pose" (touching my head to my feet) feeling blood flow near my belly button. This is what I was feeling again, now as an adult, though I was not on my belly.

I closed my eyes trying to concentrate on the pulsation as my nurse, Jill, adjusted my monitors. I opened my eyes as the doctor rushed in. Just then, I felt a rushing sensation, as if blood were surging from my abdomen into my chest. It felt as though my blood had been shot from the barrel of a gun. My heart pulsed as though I were running for my life. Gasping for air, I lurched to a sitting position.

Just then the doctor asked how I was feeling. I told him I was feeling incredibly anxious! On the monitor, I was in tachycardia and my heart was beating over 180 beats per minute. My heart became irritable and began to randomly kick off extra beats, making me feel light-headed and weak. I couldn't focus and just felt awful. I remember thinking, Just close your eyes and it will all go away. Needless to say, the doctor stopped the medication and I eventually calmed. Within those few minutes, which seemed to last for hours; I felt I had cut a lifeline. The very medication that could ensure me some quality of life while I waited for my new heart had failed. In essence, so did I. My ego was shot and I worried about what would happen to me from here.

As I sat that evening alone in my bed, I reflected on the day's events, realizing that if my heart had continued beating at the rate it was during that event, my defibrillator would have engaged. Thank God it didn't, I thought, I am afraid of that thing!

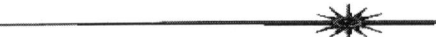

My defibrillator was implanted just three weeks after Chris and I were married. I had met with Dr. Spangenthal for my annual follow up and we had discussed changes in the insurance standards for implanting defibrillators. Even though I had not declined significantly at the time, I qualified. He explained that new studies revealed that cardiac patients with an ejection fraction (the percent of blood sent out of the heart when it contracted) less than 30%, had a 50% higher risk of fatal cardiac event. I opted for being proactive and had it implanted, but was afraid of the "punch it packed," should it go off. I was told it would be comparable to being "kicked in the chest by a mule!"

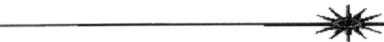

My thoughts were interrupted by another visit from the medical team. I was learning that seeing them outside of doctors' rounds was problematic. Just when I thought things couldn't have been more disappointing or frightening, I learned there was always room for more. My P.A. line kept "dampening" or wedging itself in my artery. It was another complication that I didn't understand. At this point I just wanted to sleep. I was physically, mentally, and emotionally exhausted.

The doctor attempted to advance the line in the my neck pulling it back to check placement. Of course, yanking on a tube planted in the vein in my neck was quite alarming and needless to say, uncomfortable. I was told that the line would need to come out if the dampening continued to wedge because the tube was actually at risk of blocking blood flow. I did everything I could to preserve the line including lying completely flat for as long as I could between trying to get enough air. Even this task was unmanageable and despite valiant efforts, it was destined; the tube needed to come out. I was starting to feel as though it couldn't get worse, nothing had gone as planned and my spirit weakened further. Each visit from each doctor seemed like a game of cards determining what the next draw would be, sort of a "wait and see" situation.

Dr. Mudge was the one who delivered the news to me that the doctors would need to meet to decide to attempt another type of medication. If I passed all of the required tests, another P.A. line would need to go in meaning another trip to the O.R., more observation, and a longer stay.

I missed my family and struggled with each change in my plan. The harsh reality remained that as I weakened, my coping skills were not only tested but evolving. With each medical twist, I became more educated and a somewhat more proficient champion of decision making.

The decision was no longer mine, the line needed to come out. I was well-informed about the procedure for removing the P.A. line and should have been strong. I was, however, a wimp when I realized the "forgotten and dreaded" bandage would be removed first. There is no way to prepare for that one searing rip. The nape of my neck was now red and inflamed with some torn skin. I felt wounded physically and emotionally.

POTHOLES

Dr. Campbell was the one to pull the line. I was asked to hum as she began to pull. Almost immediately, I got a stabbing pressure in my chest as if I had been stabbed dead center into my sternum. It was one of those knock the wind out of you pains and it felt like someone was trying to stab me with a knife that was too dull to penetrate. Of course, I said a silly thing, "That hurts!"

Perhaps because I didn't yell, the doctor's response was equally flat: "It shouldn't," she said. I blocked out my surroundings to process what I heard the doctor say, I thought, *I didn't hear her right. I'm having pain and being told I'm not supposed to...what?*

I remained silent the rest of the procedure and curled up like a wounded puppy trying to lick my wounds.

Later, Cricket stopped by. I asked if the P.A. line could've pulled on my defibrillator wire causing the pain. She replied, "Perhaps, but the ventricles are very fibrous and it may have torn some heart fibers as the tube came out of your body."

Trying to recover my sense of humor, I yelled, "EWWW!" It seemed more painful after hearing that! I later added this moment to my list of learning experiences: patience and perseverance.

My testing came back showing some decline in my cardiac function, but I was very proud of the seven minutes I put in on the exercise bike! The numbers began to mean very little: a cardiac index of 1.8 and an ejection fraction of 20%, my left ventricle was very sluggish and both my tricuspid and bicuspid valves were leaking. When they listened to my heart the familiar "lub dub" had now been replaced with new sounds. My heart was now irritable and the EKG showed negative changes. I think my heart wanted to go home!

Dr. Mudge got the task of telling me that the team decided they were causing me more harm than good and felt my heart needed to recover before another drug trial. I was sent home and I was scared: scared to be sent home without the medication but not sad to be going home! I was told not to worry because, "If anything happens, your defibrillator should kick in!" I was not reassured!

Once I mentally adjusted, I was happy to be going home. I reflected on how lucky I was to have this opportunity to get mentally and spiritually well, and how fortunate I was to have great family and friends surrounding me. I still felt fairly good most days and told myself, "I'll take it!"

Reflection:

It is amazing how much your body can endure physically and mentally before it seeks an escape plan or alternate mechanism of self-preservation. What is amazing is that these skills are learned through the trial and error experiences of your life. I was fortunate to have developed a sense of humor when dealing with situations as they arose and the ability to listen before I reacted. Often I needed alone time to process information that I had been given and had to sort my emotions out of decision. Now I found that trust led the way.

Being dependent on others was disheartening, but once I was able to get past my anger I realized that I needed to concede and allow others to help me. Looking back I realize how incredibly important faith, family, and friends are. In fact, I kept three items at my bedside to remind me of that very connection: an angel pin, a necklace, and a worry stone. Once I realized that I was not infallible, these mementos were frequently held within my hands when I became weak to remind me I didn't have to do it all myself. I was like a hot air balloon that required the strength of many people underneath holding onto me to prevent me from flying out of control.

As often as I think about them and pray thanking God for them, there are no words to adequately express the impact my family and friends played in my life, my illness, and recovery. I am eternally grateful that God has placed them here. I hope that in my lifetime I am able to identify opportunities somehow to reciprocate. I once worried about how I could ever repay the debt of gratitude. Since then, I have realized that what matters are those random and routine acts of kindness. They are the best contributions I may ever leave behind.

"There is a deep peace that grows out of illness and loneliness and a sense of failure. God cannot get close when everything is delightful. He seems to need these darker hours, these empty-hearted hours, to mean the most to people"

-Frank Laubach

Chapter 3

A Recovering Agonal Heart

The heart is the life force for the body. It transports blood into your organs, tissues and your every cell. It delivers oxygen and nutrients, removes carbon dioxide through the lungs, and other toxins through the kidneys and liver. It has an independent as well as an integral purpose. Your heart functions the way people should in life, pouring goodness in and forcing negative toxins out. It functions the way your parents should, nourishing your development and protecting you from harm.

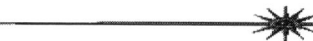

I believe now that I know why God gave me a defective heart, but there are still times when I wished He had not. For me, the memories can be painful. The truth is, I knew I had a broken heart before any physician was aware. A broken heart does not need to be diagnosed, it can be felt.

My mother's past haunted her. The loss of her mother, the abuse of her father, her insecurities, all led her to flee. She was rebellious and set out to prove she was her own person neither caring about nor needing anyone. As valiantly as she tried to be tough on the outside, an insecure, lonely child lie within. Her lack of ability to connect was as contagious as the chicken pox virus and equally as capable of later returning in life disguised just as shingles can. For us her Dad's inability to nurture and love repeated itself in her generation and in mine.

My Aunt Rita would tell us how mom would smoke cigars in public as a young teen, an act considered taboo in the late 1950's. She drank and made her presence well known in their home town. It mortified my Aunt Rita who seemed to always get caught in the middle of mom's escapades. Mom spoke her mind and pulled no punches. She had spunk and she made it known that no one could hurt her! As Aunt Rita would cry, sucking her thumb, mom would reassure her. "Don't worry Rita, they didn't hurt me," she would say.

At 16-years-old, mom became pregnant and married a boy named Fred, doing what was considered proper. A repeated pattern of abuse had ensued and my mom was able to divorce him before the baby was born. Fred attempted to harm mom. He held her at gun point and punched her in the abdomen. Mom held true to her convictions (even in 1960), and was heard, allowing for divorce. She seemed to set a precedent! She gave birth to my sister Patti, September 10, 1960, becoming a single mother, wounded prey, vulnerable to fall victim. The pattern of children outside of wedlock was followed by bad marriages out of necessity. Divorce began with her and followed me.

She met my father, Angelo, who was a father figure to her, mature and seasoned in life. The thirty years separating their age did not prevent her from becoming his third wife. He adopted my sister Patti as his own, closing the door to their past. Though I have a great deal of respect for what I know of him as a person, a professional, and my father, I wonder about the families he left behind and how his relationship with my mom was perceived.

I was told he had six children and several grandchildren from his previous marriages, all around the same ages as my sisters and I. While in high school, I met some of them accidentally making the connection with our last names. I was in the same grade as Sue, but Elaine, Kylie, and Kathy were also close in age. They would have been Angelo's granddaughters (*my nieces*). I would sometimes look at them trying to see my past, connect to what I didn't know, yet somehow felt it was taboo. We would joke that I was their aunt and I became "Aunt Linda."

Dad had a son, Michael, from his second marriage to Lucille, whom I called Aunt Lucille. The dynamics seemed odd and no one really talked about what exactly was going on, but we lived with her at intervals and she and mom got along well.

Michael was older than I and had fiery red hair that matched his temper and he always seemed to be in and out of trouble, especially with drugs. Perhaps his problems were the result of an absent father that worked out-of-town or maybe just lack of stability. I guess I don't understand at what point a child faces adversity and makes the conscious choice to make bad decisions. Whatever was missing from his life was significant enough for him to take his life while in prison.

When I was 12-years-old, the phone rang. "Hello?" I said. The unknown voice proceeded. "Hello, you don't remember me but I am calling to let you know that your brother Michael is dead."

"Dead?" I said. "Was he sick?"

"No honey, he hung himself in his prison cell by using the elastic band of his underwear. I'm sorry to have to tell you the news."

"O.K.," I said, "thanks for calling."

I have to admit I was a little bewildered. Who makes this kind of a phone call to a kid and do they ever think of the repercussions it may have? However complex it all seemed, in the short time my parents remained in each other's lives, I had a home. Now with both of them gone, the past had been that: the past.

Mom went on with her life after my father passed away. She went through the motions of life, never seeming to be emotionally connected. I do recall moving from Aunt Lucille's into a cottage with mom's new boyfriend Wally. Mom used her money to remodel the house, making it into a home able to accommodate three children. Wally and mom never married; trust seemed to be lacking. Perhaps mom was unable to give love unconditionally or perhaps her history didn't allow it. Remembering now how mom moved through life, I am sure I learned my art of distraction from her. None of it was clear, boundaries blurred. Keep busy though, and the emptiness goes away for the moment.

Many nights mom would take us out of our warm beds because of an altercation between her and Wally that usually surrounded alcohol or infidelity. Sometimes we'd visit Aunt Lucille, other times we'd be whisked off to visit Wally's family in Pennsylvania. It wasn't uncommon.

"We're taking a road trip guys!" she would tell us.

I liked the excitement of loading our blankets and pillows into the car, feeling the cool nighttime breeze on my face, and seeing the stars. Mom drove an Oldsmobile convertible, in red of course, with white leather seats. To me it was an adventure that represented opportunity for change; a new bed, a new place, and a new beginning. I learned that life lesson from mom, not to attach myself to anyone. Mom always seemed to come back to Wally though.

In 1971, nine chaotic months surrounded mom and our family in death. Her brother Joseph and her sister Joanne became extremely ill. They had problems with their hearts, experienced fainting spells, periods of weight gain, and shortness of breath, and hospitalizations all leading to their demise. After that trying time, my mother became an advocate for the family consumed with calling distant relatives in Scranton, Pennsylvania, to discover puzzle pieces that might help save lives. She even began to contact medical authorities, including Cornell University, to evaluate this cloud of death.

In the years surrounding this time my cousins Dawn, Joey, and Denise had also died. My Aunt Alice (my godmother) had lost her husband (my mom's brother, Uncle Joseph) and three children to the fatal disease. Looking back, I cannot imagine the burden branded into her soul. I truly don't know, as a mother, how you recover from that?

POTHOLES

Mom found comfort in the arms of my Uncle Lee (her deceased sister Joanne's husband) and they were married. I was just 9-years-old. All I know is that I was asked to take a bus pass to my uncle's house after school, and then mom announced my uncle as my new step-dad and that this was my new home. I wondered what happened to Wally. I barely had the opportunity to get acclimated before they purchased a home together. Once again we were shuffled off and the word home became absent of meaning.

At the age of 30, my mom was in her third marriage. We moved three times while I was in the third grade confirmed by three class photos as the result of mom's tumultuous and failed relationships.

When mom left Lee and returned to Wally I was disappointed. We had a nice home, and we had met great friends. I believed marrying Uncle Lee was a desperate attempt for love and stability, built from her fear of dying too. Yet while she sought security, she discarded ours. I suspected she knew more than she let on to the rest of us and maybe she felt Uncle Lee was that someone that would take care of her too.

Uncle Lee was a loving husband (to my Aunt Joanne) especially when she was sick with "the family illness." He worked, maintained the house, and took care of her kids (my cousins, Susie, and Michael) all while attending to her every need. I think Mom saw him as a protector and felt she could model their loving relationship. I know mom just wanted to be loved and taken care of. Her inner child continually yearned for more.

I believe Uncle Lee and Aunt Joanne were "soul mates" and he never seemed to get past her death. Mom didn't seem to be happy and their marriage ended as quickly as it began. He went on to marry several more times in his lifetime and I believed he searched for a love that would be unrequited.

Mom was sometimes irrational and impulsive repeating some of the abusive patterns of her childhood. When we misbehaved we were punished, sometimes severely. She seemed to enjoy the power of instilling fear within us and it was difficult to get solid footing on what was right or wrong.

I recall one time when she found her stereo was broken and how she interrogated us. One by one she pulled us aside beginning her process. Despite how young we were, we wouldn't tattle on one another regardless of the consequences Patti broke it and we all knew it, but no one admitted to it. As punishment mom said, "Fine, if no one is going to tell the truth, then you will all be punished. Go out into the yard and search for a beating stick." It was kind of a game I guess, one all too familiar. We knew not to bring in one that would break or be too thin, this would anger her more. We learned to avoid ones that were too green that would act more like a "switch." Perhaps it was a psychological game for us to think through what we had done wrong or even one to allow her time to calm. I don't know. It was just one more mechanism that dulled our emotions. Today, we laugh about the things we did to "prepare for a beating," knowing we never really understood what that meant.

POTHOLES

At times, mom was fun-loving and we'd do things with her and my cousins, Michael, Jimmy, and Billy. I loved that person. She loved to take "the boys" whenever she could and seemed to prefer their company. I guess she thought girls were more maintenance and maybe we were.

I recall all of us loading up the car and going to Crystal Beach, an amusement park in Canada. She never spared a penny and we ate, rode, and laughed till our hearts' content. Our last ride was called the "Himalaya." We all stood in line together to take our last thrill ride of the day. The carts swung freely as they propelled around the circle and the music blasted. Mom loved loud music, loved to laugh, and loved to sing. These were the qualities I inherited from her. On the ride she bellowed louder than the music and I could hear her calling out to all of us. It had been a perfect day.

As we all began getting off the ride, we were laughing, reminiscing about the day. Mom was last and as we approached, one of the carts swung into my mom's thigh with a force so severe, she buckled at the knees. I never saw my mom weakened by anything: ever. She called to the boys for help, something my mother never did. She didn't cry, she didn't whimper, and probably wouldn't have called out at all if it weren't for the broken femur which prevented her from bearing her own weight. It was an unexpected turn of events, and an odd end to what was a wonderful day.

Mom had little tolerance for things that slowed her down, and I'm sure I learned that behavior from her. It's also probably one of the reasons she wasn't thrilled with raising children. Often she did things other people would consider drastic to prevent inconvenience.

When I was 8-years-old, mom went to the dentist because she had a toothache. When she got home she called out for us throughout the house. I yelled, "I'm in my room!" At the time I was sitting on the floor intently playing with my "color forms." Mom opened the door saying, "Linda Mc Gee!" She called me by the nickname she often used for me. I looked up in horror and burst into tears! Her entire face, the only face I had grown to trust, was swollen and distorted. Her dark, hollow mouth housed nothing but the swollen, bloody crevices that once held her teeth. She had them all pulled so that she would never again have to endure a toothache! We ate baby food for the next few days. My favorite was banana.

Maybe as a parent the shock value was worth sending her child into refuge, I don't know, but I became instantly afraid of her at the time, unable to face this person who looked like a monster. I was young, impressionable, and simply too insecure to even try to understand. It was hard not to wonder what she would do if I became too problematic.

I have come to suspect that her willingness to simply rid herself of anything that caused her pain or discomfort may have been what led to her demise. Not too long after her mouth healed and she began to wear dentures, my mom also began experiencing problems with uterine bleeding. I was too young to know anything about that (thank goodness, I would probably have been traumatized!), but I learned she was recovering from an elective total abdominal hysterectomy! Her motto became, "If it causes me trouble, dispose of it!" Perhaps the clot was a complication from that surgery or perhaps it was God's way of ending her turmoil forever.

My father's death was a sad blur. My mother's was not. It remains a vivid memory that began with a beautiful vision of the type of love that should be shared between a mother and a child.

It was a great night and mom and I were lying on the couch together where I felt wrapped up in her love and embraced with her warmth. We were playing a game that she created to teach me how to use my new padlock for school. Mom had ordered her favorite treat, a sheet cheesecake topped with blueberries, cherries, and pineapple to be delivered right to the door. Back then the "Dew Drop Inn" delivered cheesecakes and pizza. It was the only interruption to my lesson in learning to memorize the combination to my lock. "26 to the right, 34 all the way around to the left, and 12 to the right," she said.

Now that I was in fourth grade I needed to lock up my gym clothes and the new procedure frightened me. We timed one another to see who could open it faster, but she kept bumping my arms teasingly and interrupting my thoughts so that it took me longer.

"Mom, stop it!" She was playing unfair and laughed jovially at me as I struggled!

That's not fair," I contested.

As frustrated as I was, I couldn't be mad at her. She was funny and her giggles resonated throughout the room. She was my mom, the pretty lady everyone loved, especially me. She was full of energy, appeared to love life and that night I felt connected, was happy, and peacefully fell asleep beside her. It was a gift from God.

Curled up and comforted with memories of love, my rest was abruptly halted when I heard a voice pierce the air. "Mary! Mary!"

My interest was heightened as I stirred in the darkness. Again I heard the familiar voice frantically calling my mother's name. I felt a painful sting rip through my body forcing me to become more alert. I listened intently, afraid to open my eyes. I realized there was something strange about the voice as it seemed anxious and panicked. I was trembling, my heart beat in fear.

I stretched, opened my eyes, and tried to focus my vision on where I was through the darkness. It was Wally, who cried out in terror. I recalled recently moving back in with him and recognized where I was. I was thankful; so far things were good for all of us. I thought to myself, *why is he still home? He should have left for work by now as he always does.*

But just as the morning silence was broken, so was the darkness, and what was left of stability in my life. Once again, I closed my eyes hoping that if I kept them closed long enough things would be okay. I pretended to be asleep as I listened to Wally dial the phone. Truth began to surface and I froze. I laid there motionless, just as my mother lay in the other room.

Within minutes, the blur began. I heard sirens piercing the eerie quiet of the house and the rustling of people coming through the door. It was like an invasion with flashing lights in reds and blues pulsing through my closed eyelids. Once I dared open my eyes, I could see dark silhouettes of emergency personnel and the occasional flash of a metal from a policeman's badge. Despite it all, there was one moment that shattered all the commotion.

Oh my God, no!" I'll never forget the shrill, bone chilling terror in my Aunt Rita's pleas. I remained paralyzed in that moment, her voice causing my heart, a heart that had been healing ever so slowly, to once again begin to bleed. I knew unmistakably my life had suddenly taken another fatal twist.

The noise calmed, people seemed to echo in the distance. I got up unsure if anyone was aware of my presence, not knowing where my sisters were. I tiptoed into my mom's room while the adults were at the dining room table; still in the dark. Mom was lying face up peacefully in her bed. The darkness continued to lift outside. The dim glow of the night-light illuminated her face. The room was painted a pale green causing her face to appear ghostly white. The morning sun seemed to struggle to break the darkness and I struggled further to understand.

To the touch her skin was cool, but the bed was warm. I did not utter a sound, but in my confusion I wanted her to wake up. I was curious as to why she was not moving, why her skin was so pale, and why she didn't acknowledge my presence. Why was this happening? I couldn't make sense of it. She reminded me of "Snow White" lying there motionless. I thought for a moment that maybe her prince would come too.

Looking back that was all she truly ever really wanted; a prince to sweep her off her feet and to live "Happily ever after." I now wonder if she were watching the turbulence from above or if she'd been caught off guard by her death and was trying to comprehend it herself. I wished I had been more intuitive then.

To be honest, I don't remember much of that day and feel guilty as to why I did not recall where my sisters were during it all. I have a glimmer of recollection of my older sister Patti storming out of the door to go to school. As she left she yelled back at everyone, "I'm not staying here!"

I could not comprehend any of it. She was leaving for school and mom was dead. Mom was dead; it was November 8, 1973. I wondered if this was what was supposed to happen.

Once again I detached myself from my emotions; I flipped on my self-protective switch and went into survival mode. It was now a learned behavior engrained within my heart, a heart now numb as if another part of it had died. Soon after a policeman escorted my younger sister Joyce and I from our home. Though he was a stranger to us, it seemed normal to go where we were asked with whomever we were told.

I do remember thinking how cool it was to get to ride in the back of the police car. We rode pressing our faces and palms against its windows. At just eight and nine years old, there was a quiet reassurance that Joyce and I shared because we had a bond like no other. Ironically, like my mom and Aunt Rita, we were like twins.

Despite me being a year older, I was tiny for my age and she was the same size as me. We were difficult to tell apart and looked like little "Shirley Temples." We had sandy blonde curls that were wound just a little too tight, big brown eyes, and creamy white skin dusted with freckles. We were often dressed alike and for the most part we were inseparable!

I was always thankful to have been blessed with a sister that I loved so much and had such a close relationship with. She made me feel loved, gave me a constant in my life and a purpose. I appreciated her presence. She was my only stability, and we took care of one another the best we could.

My mother's wake and funeral was the first I ever attended. It was like a bad dream, but at least we were invited. We were too young to understand this ritual or the long term impact it would have. There was no other parent to pick up the pieces and at that time our destiny lay void and undefined.

At 31-years-old my mom lay motionless in a copper-colored casket with ivory colored satin pillows, surrounded by flowers. The room filled with faceless people I didn't recognize, vibrations of conversation, some laughter, some wailing, and of course many tears. The smell of alcohol and cigarette smoke wafted throughout the room, something I was all too familiar with.

I tried to follow the lead of others. I knelt in front of the casket, not knowing at all what to do. I touched mom playfully poking at her bare arms. She was cold, her skin hard now and her rich, long brown hair was combed to one side. It spun into a single gracious curl that draped the front of her gown. *She never wore her hair like that,* I thought. *Why was she wearing this mint green gown?* She was dead! She was dead, just like my dad and never coming back. I did not want to remember her like this, in a box, lifeless, painted with makeup and bright, blood red lips. I was angry with her and paralyzed with guilt.

I carried an exhausting secret for years. I was convinced mom died because of me. I believed I killed her with my thoughts! I couldn't forgive myself for the dispute we had and what I said to her shortly before she died. Mom and I were talking at our dining room table. I had shared information with her that I learned in school about smoking and cancer.

"Mom," I said, "we were shown movies with the pictures of black speckled lungs from people who had died and people who had holes in their throats to talk and breathe that had survived. Please stop smoking; I don't want you to die!"

"No," she said.

I was baffled. How could she refuse? I was pouring out my heart to her, afraid for her life. I had made the connection of everyone in our family dying to cigarettes! I wanted her to do everything she could to be alive! I was angry.

"You are going to die too!" I yelled.

"So?" she retorted.

"Then I won't come to your funeral!" I yelled at her.

"Then don't." Her voice was stern, but cool and careless. I remained quiet knowing better than to continue. I had lost. Yet a few weeks later, she was gone.

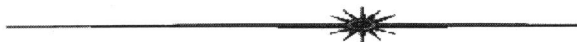

Recalling that conversation, I knelt at the casket afraid of what I had done. It echoed hauntingly in my mind, yet here I was forced to be there at her wake against her wishes. I was afraid she would come back to punish me!

The funeral took place on a cold November morning. Our breath could be seen in the crisp winter air. The sun shone brilliantly and the snow dusted ground crunched under our feet as we walked through the cemetery. I didn't cry; I was strong and brave my bubble intact. I thought, *that's what people want to see.* I held it all in.

Still, to this day there are moments, moments that resonate over and over in my mind. As that casket was lowered into the ground, I watched my Aunt Rita throw herself over the top of it. She hysterically pleaded with God. Please God, take me too!" she sobbed.

I felt confused and alone as I sat trembling. Perhaps it was the crisp morning making me shiver, but more likely overwhelming panic. Time stood still, and then suddenly, I was whisked away.

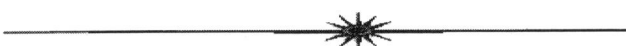

It would be many years before I would understand. Still, this pain did not compare to what was to happen next:

it was the pain of rejection that had the power to cripple me for the next years to come.

My sisters and I found ourselves sitting in the courtroom groomed like pets. The symbolic second part of my heart vacant with the loss of our second parent left us little to hang on to. We became wards of the state; custody granted to Wally.

My perception was that we were deserted by our parents and now not wanted by my Aunt Rita, my mother's twin of all people! Even as a little girl this did not seem right. She should've been our only hope, our lifeline. I was too young to understand.

Reflection:

As an adult, I have recognized that the pain of loss should not be permanent and truly our lives are not unique. We all have a story, a different path to follow and a process of lessons to endure. When we grieve, we miss the ones we love on a physical level. In a healthy process, the loss becomes less traumatic over time.

When I was younger, I felt I was able to cope better than most because I was unable to fully develop connected emotions. I was able to separate myself upon recognizing harmful emotions, and then set them aside. On some level, I felt this was a blessing that would help me process my feelings to a point where I was better equipped. For me not knowing what a parent represented over a lifetime was safer; not allowing myself to experience trust or emotions saved me from self-destruction.

POTHOLES

I've learned that the actions of our families become the foundation we use to model ourselves. Through our families, we develop and define ourselves and establish patterns. It is difficult, if not impossible to separate what is healthy from what is not.

It wasn't until I became a parent that I fully understood the significance of healthy, loving bonds that we innately develop from having our own children. Like my parents, I was blessed with three children. To me, each child was uniquely beautiful and unconditionally loving in return. I am saddened to feel that possibly the greatest loss for my parents were that they did not have the opportunity to experience the love and stability that I have enjoyed with my children. (If only they had been able to sit still long enough to have appreciated me!)

If my mother was alive today and I could give her one gift, it would be the knowledge to know that the greatest love of all is the love of God and the love of self. As difficult as it is to fully understand, if you can step out on faith fully believing and trusting in your faith, the rest ultimately follows.

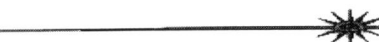

"Grieving what isn't possible in life, we eventually become free to celebrate fully – with thanksgiving, delight, and sense of wonder – what is."

Ann Kaiser Stearns

Home is Where the Heart is:

The heart is a pump made of specialized cardiac muscle. To perform well, it needs to be taken care of: fed properly, exercised regularly, and maintained in a healthy environment. If its needs are met, it thrives, functions effortlessly and becomes incredibly effective. I believe this would also be true of any person alive; if his or her basic human needs are met, he or she too will thrive. Personally, I think it is a journey in itself to recognize the difference between wants and needs as well as understanding that God gives us only what we need.

The stronger the heart muscle, the less work it has to do to meet the demands placed upon it. The well-supported psyche is also healthy and strong. These things can be cultivated. It is true that there are many factors that can upset this balance; stressing the heart or weakening the individual. Some we can control, others we cannot. Genetic disorders, race, and heredity are out of our hands and my family's heart condition falls into this category.

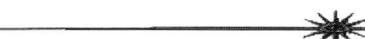

On March 1, 2009 I returned to the hospital for another medication trial. I was fortunate to have had another quiet, uneventful month at home prior, learning how to nurture myself and how to be a patient. I developed a wellness routine with music, stress reduction, and some yoga. My heart had little to offer, so each healthy deep breath was appreciated for the value it brought into my body.

I learned to love the sunshine that allowed enough warmth to enjoy brief walks with the dogs; walks that became dramatically shorter and intolerable, yet I looked forward to them appreciating each step I could take. Simple things like walking to the mailbox became planned activities, but I clung to them as uniquely mine.

Being at home on the transplant list placed me as a "level 2" candidate meaning that my acuity or complexity level was less than those requiring hospitalization. I wondered how much longer I would endure at home without an adverse or even fatal event and prayed that God would continue to allow me some dignity as I grew sicker. Unlike my mom, I did not want to die at home for my children, Chris' boys to find me. I feared history repeating itself.

I understood the transplant lists to be like time in a bank instead of money. With this bank, however, the sicker you were, the more secure your funds were and the better the interest rate. Level 2 is the least desirable account or the lowest on the priority list for an organ, while the "1 B" and "1 A" lists are more desirable. My life had come to a slow crawl on the list 2 and I feared what would need to happen to move upward. It was a numbers game for time as well as the "luck of the draw" based on blood and tissue type, and body size.

Now back at the hospital for a scheduled visit and testing, I would trial a second medication called Milrinone (a drug similar to the Dobutamine) through a new P.A. line. This visit had the same rules: trial the med, and if all goes well, go home on it with nursing services while waiting for an organ. I had begun to think of it as an organ now instead of a heart which depersonalized it from belonging to another person.

I still struggled with that. In fact I would have awful, vivid dreams about mass casualties or car accidents in which I would be walking through the destruction looking at victims as if I were shopping for my chance at life from the tragedy. Despite not knowing them, in my dreams one of the victims would have to die and be a match for me. I would walk away from it thinking, *It's all senseless death.*

Yet here I was again at the hospital going through the motions to save my life unsure that this was truly God's plan. I met with the chaplain Katherine, and we talked about hope. It was a term I didn't fully understand. Hope to me is the belief that something you wanted badly could happen, yet had the potential not to. It was an uncertainty that I guessed fit the situation.

As a patient in the hospital I felt stripped of my daily pleasure. I was not able to walk the dogs or walk to the mailbox: silly, simple things. I knew the drill as if I were in a military camp; seven to ten days in the hospital, another P.A. line in, no showers or bathroom use until the line came out. It was my very own game of "Survival," and I envisioned the bed as my island. I was dreading it, but looked forward to my light at the end of the tunnel. I believed I was fortunate. Unlike other patients who remained hospitalized, I was well enough to return home.

Still convinced I wasn't sick enough to be there having been sent home previously, I believed God had different plans for me at the time.

Prior to this admission to the hospital, we had learned that Chris' broken leg had not healed properly and the femur was not adhering to the stability rod. He had noted gaps in the bone causing continued suffering and increasing pain. Walking remained laborious for him. I could see the strain in his face and hear his dull, muffled groans as he attempted to complete day-to-day tasks. He refused to utilize pain medication because his body had become dependent on the Lortabs after his surgery following the snowmobile accident. Withdrawal for him had been torturous. He vowed never to go through that again.

He needed surgical intervention. I believed God was giving me this time to care for him. I prayed for the strength to care for him at home when I returned home and before I would again be hospitalized. We scheduled his surgery for March 19, 2009 with the belief I would be able to be there for him. I wanted desperately to be there for Chris at least this one last time before my surgery. I loved him that much.

For me, I was now on a medication that seemed to work miracles. I felt wonderful for the first time in months. I had incredible mental clarity as if I could conquer the world.

"How are you feeling?" Dr. Desai asked.

"Amazing!", I told him.

"That's the beauty of these medications; they make you feel well while you are waiting, but remember you are not. Your heart is the same sick heart, just working better on medication," he said.

Within a few days the doctors decided to add the Dobutamine back in knowing I tolerated it at lower doses. They titrated slowly, I kept my fingers crossed and I did great! In fact, I felt that if I weren't attached to all that equipment, I could have run a marathon. I felt that good and began to get mischievous.

I learned to navigate my room with my "leash" of I.V. tubing hanging from my neck and arms coupled with the lead wires for the EKG. I was connected to a myriad of monitors, entrapped almost like a fly in a spider web. I became pretty creative with the position of the furniture and even impressed myself with my new found agility as I jumped over electrical cords and equipment to get to the bedside commode. Ah yes, the commode, it was quite a lesson in vanity, but a heck of a lot better than using the bedpan!

My sense of humor also began to return as I would end up laughing as a child might, at the simplest things. In fact, I giggled one day when the doctor listened to my heart because her stethoscope stuck to my chest from all the sticky pads of the EKG wires. Her face was priceless as she carefully peeled it off, but of course I was easily amused!

I found it a little tough to sleep with all the wires dangling from my body. The plastic stockings (wrapped around my legs to promote circulation) also kept me from a sound sleep. Each time they inflated, it felt like someone was grabbing my legs which made me increasingly aware of sweat I created beneath them. It was quite disturbing! I laughed at myself as a nurse remembering my motto, "If a patient was crabby enough to have complaints, he or she was better off than one who couldn't." That was me, an inwardly crabby, but compliant-filled patient!

Day and night the nurses came in hourly to do cardiac readings. Of course some tried to be courteous and not wake me but I preferred they make enough noise to alert me of their presence. As a human being (not just a cardiac patient) I found it worse to be startled when I opened my eyes to someone standing at my bedside. In fact it felt a bit creepy!

Some days were more difficult than others. I was incredibly grateful for medical technology and the medications which gave me some quality of life. I was certainly happy to be alive. As each day passed I looked forward to going home and one last effort at being a wife and mother. Deep within myself, that internal nudge told me time was drawing near and I would soon need to give in. I felt in control for now, but not for long.

Soon, Dr. Stevenson stopped by my room with news I was not prepared for. She said, "It's time to plan to stay in Boston."

I think I went into shock because I hadn't anticipated this conversation at this time; not this soon. I guess I wasn't aware of how sick I was, or had simply denied it. It was safe for me, I guess, not to have processed the gravity of my symptoms. They say "Ignorance is bliss," and I found it to be true. Not knowing or accepting the role of a "sick" patient had psychologically been a life-saver.

However, it only took a few moments for anger to hit me and take over. It crept into my thoughts like a flu; without warning and with deadly intensity. My plans to take care of Chris were shattered and I felt I had failed him. I was powerless to do anything about it! I didn't even know how to begin to process the fact that I was no longer in charge and I hadn't prepared for that. My mind spun: I didn't say goodbye to my family or anything: *I could die here*, I thought!

After wallowing in self-pity a few moments, reality then kicked in and I realized I was spending way too much emotional energy feeling sorry for myself. I knew that I had to do what was needed to get me through the transplant process and reunited with my family including my children and grandchildren. So, with the support of my family I switched gears and began to organize a plan to manage it all. After speaking with a few folks, it seemed we could make it happen.

Isn't it funny how I thought I even remotely had control? I didn't! Things began to happen whether I was involved or not and it took me a long time to realize that life would go on with or without me. At the time though, it helped me cope in a situation in which I felt the rug had been pulled out from under me. I survived and so did everyone else. Through faith and many tears I got through one of my first emotional hurdles before falling asleep.

The next morning when Dr. Stevenson came in I was prepared to move forward. "We have a change in the plan," she said. My heart dropped when I got new information regarding my continued care. "You have antibodies in your blood that could prevent you from becoming an organ recipient. In fact, there are seventy-three. We will be forwarding your results to an immunologist for review, but at this point we may be forced to remove you from the list until we can attempt to remove them. We use a process called plasmaphoresis." She went on to explain it was similar to dialysis. I wasn't exactly sure what that meant, but it didn't seem good. There was a grave look on Dr. Stevenson's face as she delivered the news.

I smiled and listened intently somehow trying to protect her from the pain of delivering bad news and protecting myself from the shock. I did not want to fall apart in front of her.

She sat beside me patiently describing a new medical plan. With this new plan, I would stay in Boston for ten more days, and then go home for a month before returning to start the process all over again. During that month at home, I would be off the transplant list (which truly scared me) but I didn't care. My thought immediately reverted to it being God's way of allowing me to go home to Chris, to be his wife in his time of need, as well as it being an opportunity to adjust to what could be my new home when I returned to Boston.

I didn't even want to process how significant these antibodies were. It was a double-edged sword because they potentially eliminated possible donors for me because of increased risk of rejection yet they gave me an opportunity to go home! My life was now in the hands of an immunologist, a specialist I didn't even know. He held my fate; determining whether or not I would remain a candidate. I couldn't begin to imagine how I would handle that type of news if I were to be rejected. Being denied an organ and rejected as a candidate: a death sentence was a blow that I was unsure I could handle; one I had never considered.

I thought I had endured enough controversy in my life and it was my turn to get better. Hadn't life been cruel enough up to that point? I couldn't envision going through the rest of my life suffering and waiting to die. It wouldn't be fair to my boys, (Chris' boys). I rationalized with God that they shouldn't lose another "mother" figure. Again, I realized I was powerless and it was not in my control. I cried extensively, realizing the possibility of a fatal outcome, evaluating how I would live the end of my life, prayed ceaselessly, and fell asleep exhausted.

Once I awoke, I accepted the task in front of me, to plan for my future. I called it "plan B." I would go home and do what I could, I would endure, and I would survive in the most dignified manner I could. I believed I could die at home as my mother had, hopefully in my sleep with minimal or no suffering. I was amazed at just how quickly I adjusted and plunged forward.

I was interested to learn that we gain antibodies through things we are exposed to including sexual partners, childhood illnesses, and through childbirth as well as exposure, in my profession, with the patients I had taken care of. How profound it was to know that there are consequences to our actions and how those consequences haunt you later in life. I wondered if every adolescent had been taught that he or she could get "bugs" from everyone he or she was intimate with and that he or she could carry these the rest of their lives, and if promiscuity would remain at the staggering statistic it is. If every one of them were handed the notion that because of their actions they could be denied medical care would it make an impression?

When all was said and done, the doctors again returned to my room with more news. The antibodies I had were not found to be significant enough to affect my ability to receive a transplant and I would revert to the original plan; staying in the hospital. By this time, that news was exciting. *Woo! Hoo!* I thought picturing myself as the character "Pig Pen" in Charles Schultz's "Peanuts" cartoon. Yes, it suited me, the child with the cloud of confusion above my head!

I used to think, *It is what it is,* but I've added *for now.* It's less definitive.

Reflection:

Being alone and learning to stay still are two of the most difficult things I had to learn to adjust to in life. Often the coping skills we develop are out of necessity and lay a foundation for patterns of response later in life. Although I would never want anyone to experience the solitude of being hospitalized over four-hundred miles from his or her family or to unwillingly endure over thirty days alone, it was the most cleansing experience of my life.

I learned to untangle and realize emotions from my childhood and understand why I responded to my familiar environment in my unique ways. By doing this, I began a ritual of self-examination during my hospitalization. At least I could choose whether or not I was going to allow an emotion such as fear or disappointment to enter my day. Often I acknowledged the emotion I was feeling, and then envisioned taking a breath and blowing it away. This allowed me to move on. I no longer needed my familiar protective bubble because now I understood the importance of insight from within, and gave myself permission to feel emotion. The key was patience, recognition, and moving forward.

For my children, in fact all children, I would like to instill the value of "taking care of your house" meaning your body, and having the strength to deny risk to it knowing you have to live there for a very long time. The body cannot be replaced, but if you take care of it, it can be remodeled and furniture can be replaced to keep you alive.

Some people refer to their body as a temple and I can fully understand that mentality. Your body is the protective coating which you are given to shield you from the elements of life. Keeping it strong and healthy is how to protect yourself from the "bugs" in the world, whether physically, emotionally, or spiritually. That could ultimately mean the difference between a good life or one lacking substance. It is a conscious choice.

"Things don't go wrong and break your heart so you can become bitter and give up. They happen to break you down and build you up so that you can be all that you were intended to be."

Charles "Tremendous" Jones

Chapter 4

Barely Beating

The pulse is a rhythmic contraction of the heart measured in beats. The synchronicity of its four chambers in harmony with one another sustain life as we all desire! It is protected by bones, a sternum, and ribs both in the front and back, then enveloped by the lungs. Nature has provided for the protection the heart needs to prevent it from injury.

A child is conceived ideally through the beauty of parents whom love one another and intend to shield their child from harm throughout their lives. I was not so lucky.

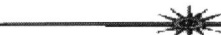

Most childhood memories are cherished as fond memories. Children are allowed to believe in Santa Claus, for the parents make it possible. During the holidays, dining room tables are filled with festive food, homes are decorated with lights inside and out, and love dwells. For me, Christmas, as for most holidays, meant visiting the grave yards of the family members who had gone before me.

We'd go to the florist with Wally (I now referred to him as my step-dad) and pick out flowers to place on my parents' tombstones. It became a ritual every holiday to wander amongst the graves, and then begin the chore of cleaning their gravestones. We started by brushing dirt from their surfaces, then we carved out debris from the engravings, and last we would pull out or kick back overgrown grass before praying. It didn't matter what holiday or what the weather-forecast, we would be there. Sometimes I would be skittish of getting mud on my white patent-leather Easter shoes or grass stains on my new dress, but to Wally it didn't matter; the job needed to be done. Once it was completed, he would send us to the car and he would break down crying.

We could see his shoulders tremble as he dropped to his knees covering his face. I guess we weren't supposed to know though because he always composed himself before returning to the car. I often wondered if he cried because the burden of custody was just too great: like grandpa. Year after year, holiday after holiday, our graveyard visits continued, making it difficult to redistribute my emotions and count the blessings I had. It all established a perfectly painful stage for my Aunt Rita to relive the darkened void of her losses

From the time I was a child and for many years forward, I watched the aftermath of loss infiltrating day-to-day events; especially the holidays. There was short-lived joy, emptiness, and many tears expelled from my aunt's Irish eyes. Through her pain, I was forced to remember the formidable memories of so long ago. I began to "unlove" her performance, unable to comprehend why reliving pain belonged among these joyous times.

I, for some unknown reason, learned to bury my grief, to detach, possibly as a way to survive. I became determined to plant seeds of hope for my future Christmases, like the ones I saw on TV and enjoyed while visiting my friends.

My friend Karen and her family seemed to have it right. Their home was filled with joy and laughter. They had a live tree that stretched ten feet from floor to ceiling tastefully decorated: amazing to look at in the dark. There were lights and collectibles everywhere. It was a true Christmas wonderland. I loved some of their traditions: singing Christmas carols around the organ while Karen's father played, going to church as a family on Christmas Eve, opening gifts afterward, and eating Italian cookies! Their holidays were a monumental celebration!

I decided that when I grew up my Christmases would be beautiful (at least the ones that I would control) and I would cultivate magical holidays. In my mind the future would implode the established patterns of sadness during the holidays.

Creating a home with beauty and harmony was difficult without an established path or proper emotional tools. The rhythm of my heart and my life was natural for me, but not what I desperately wanted. Loss was so common and it was our norm, so to me the true meaning of Christmas was not about birth and celebration which was already scarce in my life. My Christmases entailed the resurrection of death and grief.

In retrospect, Wally taught us to honor my parents by visiting their gravesites, but while his actions outwardly appeared as respectful, he took much more. He had slicked-back, jet black hair, high cheekbones, and deep set brown eyes. His distinguished features were a contrast to the ugliness within him. He wasn't the type of person whose authority you were comfortable with questioning and I doubt there could be words that could have protected me.

Wally, God awful Wally, was a man who appeared outwardly to be a knight in shining armor, one who rescued children and provided a home, yet he had a dark side; sinister intentions. It was ironic that a man in his position, receiving monetary compensation to raise children, could harbor such ugliness. He was capable of carving out your heart, and that he did. I accepted it as normal, accepted it as truth, for I was so young in my spiritual development, I understood only the lack of protection that I should've had if my parents were with me. Those were the thoughts that would accompany my tear-stained pillows.

Life with severe physical, emotional, and sexual abuse is never acceptable yet I convinced myself that I should be grateful to him for keeping my sisters and I together and not with strangers. It offered some semblance of stability. Maybe, just maybe, I perceived the abuse as the price tag. Why should I have thought any differently? Society thought he was wonderful, why shouldn't I?

Admittedly, the years of abuse did not cut as deeply as the inability to comprehend why my Aunt Rita did not seek custody of us. I believed she was the one person who I felt I should've been able to count on then, yet she offered little hope. I was too young to understand, but wish someone had at least tried to explain. I just wanted her to try. I wanted the words, "Blood is thicker than water to apply." I wanted someone to whisper the words, "Life in this family is less than perfect, but we are in it together."

Aunt Rita did what I called "spot checks," stopping in regularly with coloring books or activities, small tokens of her love, I guess. I enjoyed them; in fact I looked forward to them. She would stay awhile then be on her way again leaving us to remain like puppies in the pound.

It took me many years to accept and understands Aunt Rita's rejection; don't get me wrong, I hold no grudges. I now believe she did what had to be done in a time of instability. Then, I perceived her lack of commitment to our family as a dull knife bludgeoning my already bruised heart. As an adult, I learned that she was afraid, atter losing her brother and sisters, that she would be the next to die from some "genetic thing" that she didn't understand. I now know that grudges are not healthy and forgiveness is necessary to heal.

I would not allow the abuse from Wally to be devastating; it was numbing and quite simply he lacked connection to us. He was not engaged emotionally which was probably better for him, no emotion, no guilt. He went through the motions of providing for us. I still find myself making excuses for his behavior. One such excuse was that he was still a single man in his thirties with the insurmountable task of raising three girls, girls that would become women, as a single parent. He was overwhelmed.

Having custody of us did not curtail Wally's partying with his friends at night, a social life that he and my mother had enjoyed regularly. I believed my life was good especially in the beginning. I knew no different. I was safe with my sisters in our home and I didn't know to ask for anything more.

After mom died Wally hired a housekeeper, Mrs. Hackemer who was a kindly older woman who had raised thirteen children of her own. Her presence was competent, calming, and offered the stability I yearned for. She was the grandmotherly type with very short sandy-brown pin curls, weary brown eyes, and glasses that slid to the end her nose when she wanted to keep us in check. She would peer over the top of those glasses, and then without a word, we froze in place. She reminded me of my doll, Mrs. Beasley when she did this. She was good at "this parenting thing," but I knew she did not love us. It was not in her job description.

She cooked large quantity well-balanced meals for us everyday which served as our food until it was gone. Her motto, "Waste not, want not," held true grit as we indulged in the same food for many days at a time. I guessed her habit of cooking for her "army of thirteen" was hard to break, so a pot, no, actually a cauldron of soup lasted sometimes what seemed like an eternity. I didn't perceive this as a problem. I was hungry and I was grateful! The new environment with her in it was predictable and structured, but not a loving one.

She gave what she was able and tolerated Wally's extended absences.

I overheard a few quarrels between Wally and her. Often he would not come home after work and she would become livid. Wally normally stopped at the local tavern where he would lose track of time. Another excuse I made for him. Mrs. Hackemer would scorn his behavior and lack of responsibility. I was all too familiar with his routine, the smell of cigarettes and alcohol on his breath.

On occasion, Wally would bring home a girlfriend or two, some I liked, some I didn't. As they came and went, I learned not to get too attached; there would be no maternal outreach. As expected with any child exposed to this, rejection from each and every one of them plagued my mind. People were either paid to care or pretended to because of their relationship with Wally. It was difficult to connect with anyone at that time let alone develop a trusting, nurturing relationship. As a result, I didn't thrive much. Instinct saw me through or I am guessing that I just winged it the best I could.

Patti attempted to take me under her wing and teach me about life. Her lessons, as valuable as they were, didn't prepare me to defend myself against Wally who was waiting for me in the basement one day. The truth is, to this day, I am not sure if she needed to defend herself also against him. Sometimes, in order to keep the normalcy of status quo, you keep secrets even from your sisters.

POTHOLES

Reflection:

Forgiveness is one of the most difficult things to give when someone has violated your trust, but is necessary in order to move forward and not get stuck. I have found that there are many challenges in life and I fondly refer to them as "potholes." I coined this phrase after hearing so many people refer to "bumps in the road." I found life to be way more complex "bumps."

To me a pothole is uncertain, leaving you more than one choice. It is dark and you can't always see what's at the bottom, how deep it is, or what you will find inside. It can be filled with water, mud, or even loose gravel; all making it an uncertain surface to step onto. Sometimes you count on blind faith to see you through and other times you need to prepare with the appropriate tools to navigate around it.

If fortunate enough you recognize an impending pothole and can control your response to avoid it: swerving around it or going over it. There are times we are distracted and don't see it coming. Suddenly, we find ourselves in a situation where we must react quickly when falling in.

In life we all have our own stories, our own adversity and events we'd prefer to keep deeply seated in our souls. Each journey is different but intended intrinsically for us. I am thankful to have been able to learn to forgive despite unfortunate circumstances. I am thankful for a sister who took time to parent me, and I am thankful for the occasional person who graced my life helping me to separate stability from chaos.

As far as my "potholes" and growing up, I often found I didn't have the navigational tools I needed, therefore I learned to become resourceful. I may have gotten my feet wet, fumbled in the dark or clawed my way around, but somehow I survived.   I fell down many times, scraped my knees and pulled myself to safety. Despite facing adversity, I grew strong as I learned from my experiences. One thing is for certain, I refused to ever again remain in the unprotected dark!

When it gets dark enough you can see the stars.

Lee Salk

Making the Best of It:

A cardiac cell has the ability to contract and relax independently when isolated. Alone it serves no viable purpose, yet when combined form the heart. The cell's independent rhythmic function combines with a complex electrical system and thousands of miles of blood vessels to create the organ system called the cardiovascular system.

People can also exist independently of one another but cannot thrive. We alone cannot procreate and alone we would cease to exist. As a species, we all have an innate need to be surrounded by others like ourselves; our family and friends. We also have a need to feel loved.

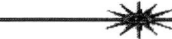

My coping skills developed slowly and have been perfected over time, yet as will happen with all of us, sadness creeps in through our pores when we are not watching. It has become easier for me to be aware of people and how they affect me. Yet, in the hospital, the emptiness that enveloped and overpowered my soul left the reality of loneliness. In the hospital, I became a child again, with only paid staff to help me. There wasn't someone there who loved me to stay by my side. The staff all became to me, paid staff. It was then that I realized the truth and accepted it. I was not given security as a child, so I find that I will regress from time to time, yet I will not allow it to define me.

The truth is God sends people to love you. Staff can get attached, there are friends that care and friends that become family. Yet, this knowledge can become reduced sometimes. I struggled sometimes with my faith when I was alone in the hospital, but it was short-lived. I just desperately wanted my family to be there, or wanted to be home with them.

My thoughts were with Chris. He had his surgery as scheduled and I was not there. I knew this was how it had to be, yet I didn't realize how hard it would be emotionally. I selfishly thought, *He is at home nurturing his leg instead of me*. I then comforted myself recognizing as life goes, plans change. I am here and he is there. The past haunts me as I sit in this hospital room, waiting for my fate. Tired now, I did wish to be the force to push forward. I wanted to be able to trust someone else to be that force. I wanted someone to be there for me, instead of being alone, but I was ill-prepared. I now was alone, again.

I grew bored, lonely, and angry. This wasn't how it was supposed to be. Being together to love, support, and care for my family in times of need is the way it is supposed to be. I kept spiraling in this world of unpredictability and I wanted things to be different. I questioned, "Was this the reason I struggled throughout my life to develop the coping skill to stand alone, separating myself emotionally only to now be reminded of that frightened child I once was?" It took a little time, yet, somehow within me, strength once again emerged forward. My heart beats strongly.

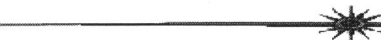

My journey has become to make life better, not only for me but for all who are reading this book. I learned how to tap into that inner core. We each have a purpose. I have found that mine is to use this trying period to educate others

POTHOLES

on overcoming disappointment, for I have faced it so many times in life.

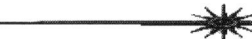

When my P.A. line was removed, I was allowed to escape the four walls of my hospital room. Carol the nurse practitioner on the transplant team encouraged me to also stay physically strong. She would caution me, "You'll be amazed how quickly your muscles weaken, and it's work to get them back." She would encourage us to walk the halls as often as we could when we didn't have a line in.

As I took my I.V. pole down the halls, I noticed I was becoming increasingly weakened with less endurance and was very short of breath. Simple tasks required lengthy naps afterward. I walked alone while other patients had families accompanying them. I mentally entertained myself by doing "figure 8's" through the hallways, checking out the floor plan and visualizing where all the doors may have led to. The I.V pole became my companion (after all it had to go everywhere I did).

No, I didn't start talking to it, at least at that time, knowing that would've been weird. I didn't want mental health issues added to my list of concerns; I was already on enough medication! Instead, I decided to have a little fun with it. Although I was physically exhausted, my mind was mentally acute and creative.

I got an idea to dress up my I.V. pole and create a friend. I used a pair of pink, brown, and white flannel leopard print pajamas my mother-in-law, Karen, bought me and then filled them with blown up hospital gloves to create a body. It took me quite a while because the non-latex gloves were less pliable to blow up, and I had very little "puff!" Next, I took a coat hanger to create shoulders and used the hook to hang my creation from my I.V. pole. I drew a face (her face) on white copier paper. She was drawn by using markers the nurses were able to rustle up. With only red for her pouty lips, black for the outlines of her face and hair, and green for her eyes, my new friend developed a striking resemblance to the character, Veronica, from the comic strip, *The Archies*.

Once I was happy with my creation, I needed to bring her to life. I shaped her head and hair by cutting her outline with scissors, then taped her together with nylon tape. This allowed me to stuff her head and neck making her 3-dimensional.

I came to a point where I needed to find a way to attach the head, torso, and extremities together. As I looked around my room, I found another perfect "Mac Giver" solution. The surgical tape left behind by one of the nurses became the perfect conduit to bring her to fruition. *Perfect*, I thought! Simply by sliding a long piece of tape doubled up for stability through her head, I had a way to hang her head onto the hook of the pole at the top, as well as a way to attach the hanger into her neck to attach her clothes for shoulders. With a few additional lengths of tape on the edges of the hangers, I created hips to hang her pants on. Additional gloves were filled to create hands and feet and were secured to the body. Her hands were taped to her body so that they didn't flail about when I moved her. Hospital slippers created a more realistic finish to her feet and I secured them to the legs of the I.V. pole. Simple finishing touches included painting her nails and utilizing tape to tailor her clothing, making her body shape more feminine.

After admiring my accomplishments, I realized I had to be cautious in naming her so that no one person could potentially feel offended. I came up with the name Bessie and because she hung from my I.V. pole, we were inseparable. My final task was a quick picture which I posted on my blog, and later introductions would follow. Though I was excited about my project, I was exhausted from the effort and allowed myself to fall horizontally across my bed for a few hours of sleep after I made her. Who else beside me would be willing to admit that I was so lonely that my IV pole became my friend?

Who else would have the courage to share this raw truth so other people could benefit, possibly finding his or her own creative way to move forward also?

As embarrassed as I find myself in sharing this raw truth with you, my hope is that you are not only able to laugh, but able to recognize my pain and my desperate, yet successful attempt to manage it. Sometimes you just do what you have to do, or like the Nike slogan goes, "Just do it!"

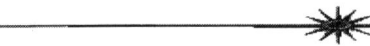

Interestingly enough, I had a few runs of ventricular tachycardia (v-tach) where my heart raced, requiring my nurse and a doctor to come check on me. This normally happens when the heart's ventricles contract independently of the atria and usually at a very rapid rate. The nurse explained, "You are in slow v-tach." I felt uniquely relieved knowing despite the abnormal rhythm, my defibrillator wouldn't fire. It was another blessing.

Because of this episode, the doctors decided I should remain in my room as a safety measure and to more closely monitor me. They decided to lower my Melrinone dose. This was to verify the medication wasn't causing the irritability. Briefly, I recalled the last medication trial that I had failed and was then sent home. I was concerned, yet too tired to worry about it. For now, Bessie and I were grounded! My stride was a little broken and my spirit beaten.

To add a nice touch to the day, both my I.V.'s infiltrated (meaning they came out of place in the veins, and the medication was leaking into my skin) causing the veins themselves to become inflamed. This in itself was a potential threat of infection; one for a heart transplant candidate that was unacceptable. I was immediately scheduled to go back to the operating room for another P.A. line.

I can't impress strongly enough how these lInes wore on my psyche, dampening my spirit. Mentally knowing that I was once again heading into another week-long period of confinement, line after line, was not only disheartening but disabling. I dreaded being dependent on others especially to meet my needs. Even more, I became downright downhearted when those that came in to care for me, with the best intentions, repositioned my few but precious possessions. I was trying to maintain some level of dignity and independence, yet simply moving my tissues or toilet paper forced my dependence.

I noted my frustration on my blog entry that day and truly enjoyed the feedback I got from my loved ones so far away. .My cousin Susie joked about getting a bag of rubber bands and shooting staff when they displaced my possessions. Her humor came from a genuine sense of understanding. She was one person who really understood what I was going through as she was celebrating her seven-year anniversary with her new heart. My friend Jane suggested a fishing pole to retrieve things myself.

The next procedure to have my new line placed reminded me of just how barbaric some medical procedures can be. I learned so much about myself, my patience, and how much my limits could be tested.

For this line they used my left jugular vein so the right side could have time to heal. I discovered the significance of my "small vessels" because they were more difficult to access and on my right side were found to be tucked behind a muscle in my neck. I never anticipated that going through the muscle would be an option.

Owwwwww! It was a painful! Afterward I was admittedly tired and very crabby; no, just plain miserable! I envisioned ripping my toenails out to feel better. The nurses were wonderful providing me with hot packs and pain medication as I needed it. Still, I refused to appear weak and refused to cry, at least in front of them. Again, my old weakness conflict was an interpersonal conflict that I don't deal with very well, surfaced.

A unique twist to my stay was that the hospitals in the Boston area were being featured in a documentary on ABC News. The series, I would later learn would be called, *Boston Med*, which would be aired in the summer of 2010. The transplant section of the hospital filled with excitement as the filming crews introduced themselves and made their presence known.

Carl was the first to interview three of my peer group and me, and we all became a part of the filming process. I was excited sharing my story, but probably more about having someone to talk to. It was a gift so badly needed and protected my sanity.

During the next few days I began to envision my experiences and emotions as a series of waves. Initially, each day seemed to bring a vicious wave that overcame me, knocking me into the sand. As the days went by, I began to transform my reaction to those blasts of waves. Instead of preparing to fight, driving my feet deep into the unstable sand, I surrendered my need to be in control. By surrendering and accepting I was awarded a series of gentle ebbs and flows instead. As I let go, I felt a new power: a comforting power. I soon began to find myself at peace.

Reflection:

There are so many things in life that can go wrong, but equally as many that can go right. It's all in your perspective. I learned that at the end of everyday no matter how good or bad, I could always find a reason to be thankful. I learned that life's needs are simple and mine were met. I had food, clothing, and a place to lay my head, along with the support of loved ones. And, I had hope. If there is one thing I hope to give back to the world it is the knowledge to embrace life's "potholes" with open arms and courageous faith. It will be those who love us, or random acts of generosity or kindness, that will see us through.

Whether it was simply talking to my family, reading an e-mail, or eating a good cookie, each day was like opening a wrapped package; inside there was always a surprise. I found joy in the anticipation. I visualized my emotions as waves that no matter how overwhelming at first, always found their way to shore. I had innate coping skills that were similar to those cardiac muscle cells: when allowed to function as intended, allowed to let go of and recognize factors which could not be controlled, the heart and I were able to find peace.

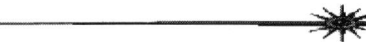

Let your hopes not your hurts, shape your future.

Robert H. Schuller

Chapter 5

A Mending Heart

When supply of blood to the heart itself is inefficient, the heart becomes stressed and irritable because the nutrients it needs are lacking. This can happen for reasons such as an occluded blood vessel or too much pressure in the system preventing the heart from getting any rest. Awareness of an existing problem occurs because angina or chest pain is experienced. Pain or pressure can occur during periods of stress or even at rest. If ignored or if the condition that caused the problem is not corrected, it can lead to a full blown heart attack (MI) in which a portion of the heart dies. If severe enough, cardiac death yields human death.

Likewise, a person has needs for survival. When they are not met, he or she may react in an unpredictable manner. Some children become innocent victims who are unable to change the circumstances of their environment. If we are fortunate, enough necessary nourishment is provided in abundance. However, children raised in a dysfunctional setting may grow to be adults who are unable to recognize how learned coping mechanisms may be unhealthy inappropriate responses in an adult environment. Without this knowledge, one could fail to develop ability to love, which may lead to a lifetime of emptiness – a different kind of pain in itself. Just as the heart will die from stress or *neglect, this too can ultimately lead to the extermination of the soul.*

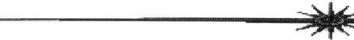

Not long after mom died, Wally met Carla. She was a gentle soul with a heart-warming laugh and was very attractive. She made a pretty mom just like mine. Her hair was long and brown, but not quite as curly. She had smiling eyes that were hidden with the dark plastic framed glasses (*indicative of the 1970's*). Although she wasn't my mother, she was probably the best thing that could've ever happened in my life. In her I saw what a mother was supposed to be.

She was divorced with four children whom she loved unconditionally and it showed. Roberta, who was her first-born and was nine months older than me, looked like a model. She had long blonde hair, streaked with highlights of color. Her eyes were blue and twinkled when she smiled. She was taller than I and thin. She was the type of person that had an outward friendly appearance and that a person might want as a friend.

Unfortunately, she yet had a confidence that was condescending and annoying. Our age separated us by a year in school so we knew many of the same people. She had a knack for playing on my insecurities, always making me feel like I was lesser of an individual, less intelligent, and less pretty. I guess typical of teenagers. We just didn't get along.

"You look like a frog," she told me one day while looking at me. "Your eyes are shaped funny," she continued. It seemed as though she derived pleasure from hurting me, and everything I did irritated her. I found her hard to like, yet was desperate for her acceptance. Despite how cruel she could be and how candidly honest she was, I wanted her to love me and I tried my best to please her. In our home she had power and I was jealous of the girl who seemed to have everything; everything but compassion.

In fact, one day she felt compelled to set me straight about life. She told me I should be grateful that their family came into my life because before then we had nothing and we were just orphans that nobody wanted. I was dumbstruck by that and grew silent. Until that moment, I never thought of myself that way, never realized anything was wrong. Her simple, effectively pungent statement weakened my self-esteem almost to the point of my pleading for her acceptance. I felt that unworthy.

I tried desperately to be a part of her life, but it seemed the price was simply too great. It left me to be a groveling slave which was humiliating. I felt that I had no place anymore and seemed to always be "jockeying for position" in my own home. Nothing was sacred, nothing belonged to me. It seemed that everything was fair game for her, but the rules only applied for her and changed as she saw fit.

Roberta was very deliberate and methodical and neither respected nor valued my personal things or boundaries. She would take my things from my room without asking, however wouldn't allow me to use or borrow hers; at least I was polite enough to ask. I developed some institutional hoarding behaviors as a result of Roberta's continuous violations of my privacy.

Knowing I would come directly to her room when I was missing something, Roberta once vacuumed her carpet so that she could see my footprints in the fiber. "Mom," she called to Carla, "I told you she comes in my room when I'm gone, see her footprints?" I was the victim yet she knew how to manipulate the truth in her favor. It was a no win situation and she was a pro at "pushing my buttons." I often wondered why everyone around us was oblivious to how she tortured me. There was no handsome prince to rescue me no fairy godmother, no one at all.

I found that if by hiding things in my room (including food) it would be there when I wanted it. *Somehow, it gave me a piece of control.* These behaviors were difficult to unlearn as an adult. The very things I admired in Roberta were things I realized I could never have; her presence in my life represented a new emotion. She was the one person I learned to hate: an emotion I wasn't prepared to deal with. She had a way of making me do the wrong thing by planting seeds in my mind. I now call them mental land mines.

There was a time she came to the house when we were eating soup that Mrs. Hackemer had prepared a large kettle of.

"Yuk!" she told us. "You eat like poor people," she continued. That simple statement made me question my life. After she left, I took the kettle into the yard, dug a hole and dumped the soup. Somehow I felt vindicated, empowered as if that single act could ease my pain; erase our differences. She represented chronic rejection, certain inadequacy in my life at the time, as she persistently feasted on my pain.

Evan was Carla's son. He was three months younger than I and was incredibly handsome, and intellectual. I loved talking to him and was amazed at how easily he learned things with minimal effort (unlike me). He had silky, straight, sandy-blonde hair, brown eyes like his mom, and great dimples that appeared as though they were deep enough to get your finger stuck in them.

In his smile was an ear to ear grin that made girls melt even after he got his braces. He was charming and respectful toward me. Our personalities clicked from the beginning and he accepted me as one of "the guys" when he needed an extra person to play football with his friends. We were very competitive with one another and I developed an affinity to being assertive, in control and in charge. Our relationship was mutually respectful, and rarely did we disagree. He was probably the first positive male presence ever in my life. Corky's (Evan's nickname) only rule was I couldn't date any of his friends, which was never a problem for me! He didn't want to be embarrassed by knowing any of the personal details, and I preferred my relationships to be kept just that: personal. The only thing he ever did to irritate me was to chew his cereal too loud…and I blamed that on Captain Crunch.

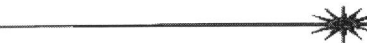

Carla's third child was Kylie who was two years younger than. She was striking with olive skin, silky, long dark hair, sharp features, and only one deep dimple. She appeared sophisticated and carried herself proudly. I found her to be intriguing yet brilliant and we had great conversations! She was well-spoken but to the point. We were pals when it came to our acrobatic classes and practiced together in the basement in the moments we could steal away from our day. I liked when she came into the basement with me so that I wasn't alone.

In our home, she got along best with my sister Joyce and that was O.K. with me. The only thing that Kylie and I seemed to disagree about was cleanliness. Both she and Joyce marched to a different drummer than I and functioned well in organized chaos. I did not!

Kylie was my first life lesson in accepting others for who they are and surrendering to my desire to change them or need to be accepted in her life. We had mutual respect and admiration for one another. It was mind boggling to me that she didn't care about her room being in disorder, as the mess represented nothing to her. To me it represented the one thing at this point in my life that was attainable; a tiny place where my things were in order.

Terri was Carla's baby and was like a fragile china doll. She had petite features with a pretty mouth, and when she smiled she was radiant. Her dimples were tiny, just like her, and she had a scar on her cheek; remnants of a mishap with broken glass as an infant. Her brown eyes appeared distant, and often she didn't seem to interact well with the other children.

When Terri started school, it was discovered that she had a significant hearing loss which made learning difficult for her, and she had fallen behind developmentally. In some ways, it made her the weak one in our blended family but in others it brought us together. That little angel we thought needing protecting became the most determined little person I had ever known and I admired her. Because of this I took an interest in her and we were the most compatible to share a room. She was a kind soul, sort of a "diamond in the rough," not as pretty as Roberta, nor as smart, but she had a beautiful presence. Her hearing imperfection taught me a lesson in overcoming adversity. She was the underdog, but once she was surgically able to recover some of that loss, she was unstoppable!

The ages of Carla's children were woven into ours. Patti was oldest, and Terri the youngest, pickling Joyce and I in the middle. Once Wally and Carla married, there were seven of us until baby Brent made eight! He was darling and I loved learning all about him. I focused on watching him grow and develop, and watched Carla closer than ever as a mom. She was a great role model. All of her children had stability and love; the ingredients to a healthy well-being. For the first time in my life, things felt like they would be alright, whatever that was to me at that time. It seemed really great to have something to rely on, and I somehow got the job of getting everybody up and out the door on time in the morning for school. This meant I got up the earliest at 6:00 a.m.; and to me it was an important job, especially when it came to pleasing Roberta. I had new siblings, a new mom, and the greatest bonus was that I also got a set of grandparents.

Carla was raised by the most wonderfully embracing couple who brought a cornucopia of warmth, generosity, and faith into my life. We didn't see them often, but when we were with them the world centered on our visit. Grandpa Isaac loved life and enjoyed talking to us. He made it seem as if we were the center of the world. Grandma Helen always baked pies (my favorite was coconut cream) and sour cream chocolate chip cookies. Visiting them was a treat just like you would see in the movies. It wouldn't be until much later in my life that I would realize how much they impacted me with their unconditional love.

    Despite some adversity, I developed a fierce need to fit in. I took pride in getting grades similar if not better than my new siblings and didn't like being second best. The dynamics of the house had changed into a deeply competitive one. It made no sense that I struggled to fit in. They moved into my house and I was the one struggling to maintain my footing. By sixth grade, even my hand writing had changed dramatically as if somehow I had evolved into someone else. I started to develop breast buds then, began shaving my legs (something Patti taught me how to do), and even had my first real crush on a boy.

    As time progressed, I realized that my new family situation displaced me from what I'd known before. Carla was now in charge. Patti, now defiant and angry pushed herself away. Joyce was not the baby sister I once knew anymore either. She conformed to her environment like a chameleon, becoming less visible. She seemed to lose her identity here; blending into the woodwork with little attention directed her way. Perhaps she just didn't care. Perhaps she just gave up or perhaps the competition was just too fierce. I began to feel isolated and resented her lack of loyalty. After all we had been through; I felt Joyce had become a traitor. Regardless, I loved her anyway. It was just a whole new world.

I now had brothers and sisters competing for a mother figure, and Patti rebelling at every opportunity. I did not know what to believe in. It became a "survival of the fittest" situation. I felt threatened and wanted to flee as my mother had once taught us!

As confusing as life may have been at this point, I will not say this was bad for me. In the face of conflict I learned to work harder to be better. I found myself resorting to my safety bubble, centering my world on me. I felt I was the only person I could count on. Don't get me wrong, I believe Carla was the best mom she could have been to me, but through my rebellious 13-year-old eyes, I could see she loved her own children more. However, I empathized with her and truly felt being a step-parent must have been an impossible task.

I recall thinking; *I would never want to be in such a situation. I don't know how I could love someone else's children.* These were the kind of thoughts that raced though my young teenage mind, a mind that didn't love itself. I rationalized other people's behavior into reasons why they couldn't love me, and likewise why I may never be able to love in return. To these thoughts now I say, be careful what you send out into the universe!

There was a clear delineation in my mind. Carla didn't know me, didn't give birth to me, and I openly despised her first-born child which made things harder. I felt incapable of fitting in or ever meeting her standards and don't understand what drove me to continue to try. It would've been easier to be the "black sheep" that I felt I had become.

I admired Carla's relationship with her children, however, and how tender she was with Brent. I admired how he lovingly gazed at her and responded to her voice. The love between them was unconditional and I wanted that! I watched in awe at how it was supposed to be and how she and Wally bonded with their baby. I wanted that too. Yet, I accepted that I was now a stranger in this house and to me it wasn't beneficial to invest too much time in a relationship with Carla or any of them for that matter. Trust was not an option.

I was envious of Carla's relationship with Roberta on many levels, but mainly because their relationship was one I felt I would never know, one I was not afforded an opportunity to have!

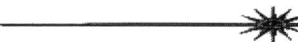

I recalled having pulled even further away after I opened myself up to Carla about problems I was having with fitting in. "Carla," I said, "I am really struggling here to fit in, and since my mom died, I don't feel at home here. I guess maybe you can't fully understand me since we have only been together a short time." To this day, Carla's words reverberate through my mind. Perhaps I was seeking affection, a hug, or some understanding, but her response cut like a razor. "Quit using your mother as a crutch!" she demanded.

I was shocked at her lack of compassion. More so, I was disappointed in myself for thinking that she might empathize with me at all. Maybe she saw it as an attempt at self-pity, but I was a 13-year-old who was genuinely reaching for understanding and love. Once again, I retreated into my bubble hating myself for opening myself up to this kind of pain.

Although it seemed cruel at the time, it turned out to be a great opportunity. I became determined to overcome and set my sites on becoming a better person. Carla helped me to realize that I needed to love myself.

From that event, I developed great leadership skills as I began to work outside the home. Initially, I babysat and had several customers. From there I took on random cleaning jobs, taught dance school, and even took a full-time position in a Youth Education Training Program (YETP) at the high school. I learned to depend on myself at a very young age.

As I grew, I recognized that outside of the home I didn't have to fight for the love and acceptance of others, it just came naturally. I developed great friendships that have lasted for many years. In fact, like my sister Patti, I found a surrogate home at my friend Karen's. We became the best of friends in the sixth grade. She was the youngest of six children, the only girl, their gift from God. We spent as much time as we could together including holidays, despite being from such differing worlds. Hers was filled with abundance and I was grateful for the overflow. Her parents (I called them Aunt Ginny and Uncle Dan) were wonderful people, and took me in as their second daughter; at least it felt that way. Her mother got me involved in the church, offered me random odd jobs to earn extra money, and held me in the palm of her hand. There I was safe, protected from the winds of my life.

Reflection:

One of the greatest gifts in life is insight. There are so many times in which we respond to our environment seemingly out of instinct, not fully understanding or knowing what the outcome, repercussions, or impact might be. Insight allows us the opportunity to react with knowledge and purpose. As we get older, it is imperative to recognize that if our childhood was frustrating, disappointing, or cruel, we can still overcome. For me, I may not have been the person receiving the positive, nurturing upbringing, but I was fortunate enough to have grown up in an environment where healthy relationships occurred with other family members and sometimes surrogate family members. It wasn't perfect, but I had an example to follow and was blessed to be somewhat safe and protected. I am thankful for the wonderful role models I did have; Carla, for what she was able to give, and especially for Aunt Ginny who saw the good in me and tried to instill good values. I have chosen to grow from my experiences to become the best I can be instead of remaining stuck in the past. Either way, I found that happiness in life becomes a choice. My friend Tony once told me, "Life is not about what happens to you, but how you respond to it." I hope we all gain the insight to recognize that we deserve a great life and that life begins with us.

Faith is not simply a patience that passively suffers until the storm is past. Rather it is a spirit that bears things – with resignations yes, but above all, with blazing, serene hope.

Corazon Aquino

Ease of Mind and Heart:

The heart responds to internal and external stimuli in the environment around it. When at rest, the heart slows down to compensate for the body's reduced needs and in turn, it too can rest. When stressed or threatened either physically or emotionally, it reacts with the potential for a "fight or flight" response, if necessary routing blood to where it is needed. Ideally we take care of our heart in its environment, through diet, exercise, and spiritual connection. It is imperative to provide the same for the ones we love. It is an ongoing evolving process.

Each day in the hospital became an opportunity to learn more about myself and to revisit my appreciation for life. From my window on the 9th floor, I could see the city awakening at dawn as the sun reflected onto my windows. Some days the sun brilliantly burst in shades of orange across the sky and others the day's last rays just streaked the skies in pink. As my world stood still, others hustled through this "walking city," among the quaint New England architecture like dubious bees. With spring came the blossoming of life. Flowers began to bloom bringing my thoughts to my flower gardens at home. I would not be there this year to reap the splendor from the bulbs I had planted in the fall. I longed to be home with my family for Easter and I was crushed when it was validated that I would not be.

While Chris continued to recover at home, I was in Boston decompensating. Despite multiple bruises from failed

I.V. sites, I was still in good spirits and able to joke about having purple (a color that never looked good on me) camouflage arms. I was again confined to my room with a new P.A. line and my four-feet of tubing, perseverating about having to endure another ten days without the pleasure of a shower, access to running water to brush my teeth, or the ability to use a real toilet. I thought about the hospital term "bathroom privileges" differently now than I did when I was a nurse. The concept that actually having a bathroom to use was a privilege not a given struck: a whole new meaning from a patient's perspective! I also recognized that I would again be isolated and alone.

Staff continued to come into my room and rearrange things to provide my care. Now, in order to ensure nothing was displaced, I'd watch them with the keen eyes of a hawk, waiting to pounce, as if they were prey. It took a lot of useless energy but I feared the repeat offenders! On one occasion, after a nurse left I realized too late that I couldn't reach the commode, the phone, or water which forced me to rely on the call bell for help.

I acknowledged their need for organization, safety, and efficiency of care, but it never dawned on me as a nurse who took care of patients what it was like to be on the receiving end of patient care. I didn't realize how positively or negatively my actions may had impacted my patient, until now.

My room was my room I now took ownership for it and I learned to take inventory of just where things needed to be so that I could maintain some semblance of dignity. In some ways it was all that I felt I had left, or at least all I had control of. Lack of control, being disempowered, made me feel as though I was reliving my sibling rivalry with Roberta. I felt beaten down and weak, finding it a difficult concept to comprehend and actually accept. So many times people echoed the words, "Let it go," yet until you are in a situation where you are brought to your knees in desperation, you can't understand the profound impact in those words of wisdom. For quite awhile I did not know how to "let go," nor what it entailed.

My social worker Kristyn came in to visit me regularly. She was a pillar of support. She give me the "stepping stools" I needed to progress in my spiritual growth and to move toward healing myself. When I looked into her eyes, I found that they were peaceful and genuine. I felt as though she could look into my soul. She was an incredible listener and had a gift for helping me search deep within myself. She offered many healing modalities, if a person was open to receive them. I had some wonderful mantras, Reiki sessions, and listened to CD's of Pema Chodron. What a wonderful spiritual growth opportunity I was afforded!

In the middle of March, the medical team was able to arrange a social networking group for those of us transplant patients that were interested. I learned that there were five transplant patients currently hospitalized just like me! Of course getting us together in one room would be fun depending upon who had a line in at the time and what space we needed for our attached medical paraphernalia. With that in mind, a date was scheduled.

I proudly walked Bessie down the hall into the patient's room where we were to meet. I was second to arrive as a man was already there in his bed. He was strikingly sickly in appearance, with pale, dusky-colored skin and sunken, deep set eyes. His voice was weak as he tried to speak and his obvious struggle to breathe told his tale. I introduced myself and waited patiently as he took a deep breath and close his eyes. His name was Steve.

I pulled up a chair and sat beside Steve's bed. I noticed that he too had a line in and while in his presence, I could sense fear. The emptiness shone through his eyes and he looked as if he'd been spooked by a ghost. He was at a breaking point having recently experienced a few recent cardiac scares requiring crisis intervention. He was desperate for an end to what appeared to be a nightmare for him. I recognized how sick he was and I automatically reached out to hold his hand. There by his side, I became fearful for his outcome, quietly acknowledging my own mortality.

The others came in shortly after. I scanned the other patients as they came into the room, organizing in my mind as to whom was the most detrimentally ill. I definitely believed it was Steve, so to ease my mind I prayed silently at the bedside that he'd get his heart before something adverse happened. My thoughts were interrupted as everyone began to introduce themselves. I snickered listening to their Bostonian dialects, and the absence of mine.

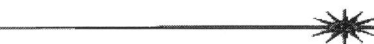

Steve was a teacher and had to overcome dyslexia in order to succeed in that role. I was amazed at the amount of dedication that it must've taken to complete that task given in the assumptions associated with a disability. I thought he was fascinating! He was married and had young children. Steve began to cry.

"I want my life back," he cried. He went on to tell us about his family and the life he longed to have back between is shortened breaths. We all choked back tears recognizing we knew his pain all too well. I was afraid for him and prayed again (this time for myself) that I wouldn't get to that breaking point. Even through Steve's physical and mental exhaustion, he found refuge somehow; and remarkably helped us too. My favorite of his sayings was: "And so it goes."

Next to arrive was Kenny. He was a Warehouse Manager in a major electronics type company. He had been hospitalized for about a month longer than I and had been ill over several years. He was our patient expert!

"I know the 'inside scoop' behind the scenes here at Brigham. You might say I'm a regular," he said jokingly.

In the dietary department, he knew how to get better food and had a separate set of menus to the elite kitchen called the Pavilion. They even prepared his favorite meal: stewed tomatoes and macaroni. "Just call and ask them to make it for you, it's delicious."

Personally I thought, *Yuk*, but he seemed so happy to share. He knew where to walk, where to sneak outside to sit in the sun, and even what not to do because he learned from his mistakes.

"Whatever you do, don't get caught outside this hospital," he said. "One day I went for a walk to sit in the flower garden at one of the other interconnected hospitals and was reprimanded."

"Dr. Stevenson was not happy and told me about it!" Kenny told us.

"You are only allowed in your house!" she told him.

We all laughed, but I had secretly thought about taking the same trip! He had great words of wisdom telling us to get out of our rooms.

"Walk when you are not tethered to your bed with a line and keep your heads held high," he said.

I really didn't comprehend what he meant by this at the time, but nodded.

Ken had seen other patients go off for their transplants while he remained behind. *Wow!* I thought at that time, never had I processed that feeling; a whole different class of rejection. Ken proudly talked about his family; his wife Nancy, his son Daniel, and his daughter Nicole. They visited often and I got to know them incredibly well as they opened their hearts to me. I watched them intently throughout my hospital stay. They were truly an amazing, selfless family! No matter how many patients went before Kenny, his goal seemed to share anything he could to make our stay easier. He became our host.

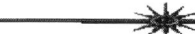

Also at the meeting, I met Kahn (I called him Dr. Ken) who was a cardiologist that was quite accomplished. The story of his illness was one of endurance and dignity. His heart beat relied solely on his pacemaker. Watching his heart monitor frightened me. I couldn't imagine this man, who had dedicated his life to wellness, a man who had run the

Boston Marathon, was at this point in his life; two massive heart attacks brought his life to a screeching halt. I admired Kahn. He was a calm soul, very accepting of his journey and very peaceful with it. He was from India and spoke with a thick dialect. As I listened to him speak, I clung to his words trying to fully understand him and to respect his cultural beliefs. I realized he was just like the rest of us. He had a wonderfully supportive family and proudly talked about his children and new grandson. His wife Surrinder was a wonderful compliment to their family.

Geoff was also a part of our group. He was registered nurse who worked with patients recovering from addictions to drugs and alcohol. Of all of us, his medical status felt like it was the most at risk. He didn't have the lifelines the rest of us had. He couldn't have a P.A. line because of a vascular problem he had, and his defibrillator didn't function. Knowing Geoff's difficulties helped me to realize how fortunate I was. My path seemed to be the most predictably normal; God has a way of helping us put our lives into perspective.

Geoff had a robust personality, great sense of humor, and very realistic outlook on life. I was amazed to hear that he was engaged and was to be married to his fiancée Sheila after he recovered. As he talked, I marveled at his positive energy and was comforted in the things we shared in common.

The last to arrive to the group was Lauren. She was the youngest of us at only 27- years-old. I acknowledged that she could've been one of my children. She struck me closest to my heart and reminded me of my daughter, Erin. I wanted to protect her. I learned that, just like me, her condition was genetic (a disorder called Dannon's disease) and she had been sick on and off since the age of nineteen. I was heart struck learning the fact that she had been sick for seven years, almost one-third of her life. It was astonishing to me and quite an eye opener. I felt guilty and her story helped me to realize from that perspective, how good I had it. I had the most ideal path among the group and actually became very thankful!

Lauren was admitted to the hospital before Kenny and they were familiar with one another. Overall, she appeared shy, but shared her enthusiasm when it was time to have her line removed that morning.

"I'm sorry I was late, but you know how great it is to shower after you get a line out. I just needed to soak and it was heavenly," she told us.

We learned that she refused to be introduced to us until she was clean. No one blamed her; we all knew how desperate we became to bask under a hot stream of water.

I sat in awe of this young spirit, a sight to behold, beautiful long sandy colored hair, fair skin, tiny little features and bright blue eyes. She was a beautiful soul with a gentle disposition who worked with children with special needs; something we both shared a passion for.

When it was my turn, I introduced myself *and* Bessie. I figured I needed to alleviate their concerns that I was from a "funny farm" or something. I saw relief on their faces as I explained that I created her as a companion for fun. I then let them know about my family situation (Chris at home recovering and me here) and that Bessie was a kind of therapy for me. I later learned that Ken and Lauren had both seen her and had previously come to the conclusion that I may have been a little odd.

"You have to be careful of those first impressions," I told them jokingly.

I think we got over that bridge early on. I shared with them that I was a registered nurse that worked in the field of developmental disabilities for over twelve years. My current position was as a nurse liaison between group homes, the pharmacy I worked for, and the medical teams. My job was to ensure good continuity of care between all parties I worked with and of course our end user, the patient.

I spoke proudly of my children: three grown children, three grand-children, and of my second marriage to Chris, and his boys. They learned that my heart problem was genetic and that two children had inherited the gene from me, which created a great deal of guilt.

I also shared with the group that my middle daughter, Erin, who had recently turned twenty-three, would be having surgery to implant her defibrillator while I was in the hospital. I held back the tears as I spoke of my daughter, afraid for her, wishing I could give her my heart. I kept the introduction short and simple because there had been so much to absorb for all of us and we were all short on energy. Kenny took a moment to add another story.

One day, the nurse moved my call light and I needed to use the commode. My room is at the end of the hall from the nurses' station so I knew that calling for help would prove futile. I picked up my cell phone and called the front desk of the hospital because it was the only number I knew.

"Hello, Brigham and Women's," the voice on the line answered.
"Yeah, this is Kenny Morrell, a patient on the ninth floor. I need a nurse in here!"
"Sir, if you utilize your call light I am sure someone will assist you."
"Well, I would do that but I can't reach it and I need to go to the bathroom!"
"O.K. sir, I will let them know," the attendant answered.
"Thanks and tell 'em to hurry, I can't wait much longer!"
What initiative! I thought hearing him tell the story. I loved his sense of humor.

What I took from that room was priceless! We were from all walks of life, all "very real" people with active lives and personal accomplishments. It was cleansing to be among "peers" experiencing the same emotions, hardships, and frustrations that I was. In fact, everyone complained about the food, staff moving things around in their room, and feeling the lack of control! Whether they appeared little frustrations or big to others, they were significant to us. We were connected and I felt I was among friends. I was comforted to know that I was not alone and recognized that in order to survive I was going to need to allow myself to need them. When I went back to my room, I had a lot of time to reflect and rest.

Some days, the routine was mundane. I was, "boringly stable," one of the doctors, Dr. Lewis told me. It was reassuring but it didn't make me feel better knowing I was still there missing my life, my husband and family whom I loved unconditionally. Their memories kept me focused on getting well, yet sometimes I felt like I was suffocating; as if not getting my basic emotional needs met. I wanted to escape! Then the synchronicity struck me. I was given a new family, my hospital family.

Little did I know, my new friends here were to become my surrogate family; an interesting twist of fate for me. They weren't paid to care about me! In fact, I was amazed to learn that in times of the greatest need I was able to develop deep, enduring relationships by simply allowing myself to reach out. I found that as I reached out there was someone on the receiving end reaching back.

Each day presented opportunities to feel and experience emotions and deep memories. I learned to recognize how my past experiences contributed to how I reacted today. I learned that, yes I was in control of my responses. In fact, there were days when I learned to recognize an emotion, acknowledge its existence, and then ask it to leave. My favorite emotion to push away was disappointment.

My ever-faithful Bessie stood beside my bed on her I.V. pole through it all, and accompanied me around the hospital when I was able to leave my room. She got a lot of attention throughout the hospital and many people approached me to ask about her. Someone even offered to buy her! Bessie often made the days interesting and occupied my time as I redressed and re-stuffed her as she needed it. In general people paid a lot of attention to her! One time I stuffed her chest a little too full and the nurses commented on where she got her breast augmentation! She was a great distraction from my loneliness.

On more than one occasion, Bessie actually startled me when I awoke at night. I thought I saw her standing at the bedside. I decided that was probably not good for my heart so I moved her to the Hoyer lift installed in the ceiling. That actually turned out to be more fun. The nurses and doctors could stand her up and move her around the room on its track. It made me laugh not only to see them play along as well as acting playfully, interacting with Bessie as if she were a puppet. They made the days a little brighter simply by being cognizant of how lonely I was. It was a simple gesture of kindness and a great little "pick me up." Sometimes we'd joke about not having a "psych" ward in the hospital for me, but we all recognized that my creativity became my coping mechanism.

On Easter Barbara surprised me with a large chocolate bunny. It was the type with the white candy eyes that were fixed as if they were afraid. I named him "Wilson" because he reminded me of the volleyball friend that Tom Hanks developed in the movie *Cast Away*. I connected with being stranded on a desert island since I was unable to leave and often tied to the bed.

A few days went by when a sense of excitement rolled through the transplant floor. Steve had been called for his heart. HIPAA laws prevented the nurses from telling us, but with all the commotion, and the ABC News crew in the halls, we all knew. The flurry of activity was telling. It was the first time the term "hope" had gained strength for me. Our group became like a team rallying for a teammate often by e-mail now since we couldn't always see one another.

Despite all the excitement, when the dust settled and the hospital quieted, we all wished it was us who received the heart; disappointed it wasn't. It was a new type of rejection at a much higher level, and Kenny's words flooded my memory, "Hold your head high."

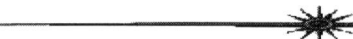

Reflection:

Coping mechanisms are developed with experience. Even in the human body, homeostasis occurs when change needs to be compensated for. Too often, when we are confronted with adversity, we become closed from embracing our experiences, or get hung up on the negative impact it may have, versus the lesson learned.

I am forever grateful for having chosen a hospital that was compassionate enough to recognize the value in patients supporting one another; creating a well-rounded approach to healing. Their insight in bringing us together was a blessing from God and a lesson for me. I realized that despite being so far from home, the definition of family is not merely only the people that you share genetic makeup with, but can also be the people you build relationships with along the way. My friend Helen believes, "People are family, our relationships are the by-products of our family, and by maintaining relationships, you in turn love all people." We have the choice to love, to care for, and stay in touch with those we love. We also can choose to support, accept and love.

My hospital family saw me through my darkest of moments. I didn't need to pretend to be anyone else in order to be accepted by them. I was able to connect with them on a personal level and trusted them implicitly.

In a period of my life where change was imminent and fear of the unknown taunted me, I was truly blessed with my hospital family. I know "there is a bigger picture," but if we don't open our eyes we will never see the opportunities that present themselves; opportunities that have been there all along. It is said that people come into our lives for a reason, a season, or a lifetime and as for my new family, I'm hoping for a lifetime!

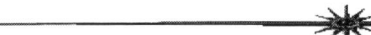

We create our lives a thought at a time. And sometimes it comes down to changing athought such as "Why did this happen to me? "There is a divine plan and there is areason for this, and my choice is to create the most positive reaction I can."
Dee Wallace Stone

POTHOLES

Chapter 6

Searching for Love on my Own

When the heart is weakened and begins to fail, doctors run tests to determine what the exact problem is. The heart muscle itself may have become inefficient as a result of other organs not working properly and causing it a greater workload. It may be the result of insult imposed through alcohol abuse, stress, improper diet, or lack of exercise. After many years of increased workload, the heart muscle itself can change, thus causing the heart to work less effectively.

We often have control over the ability to improve our cardiac health simply by changing our lifestyle or even adding medication. With proper care and follow up the heart can be managed for many years yielding a healthy, productive, and fulfilling life. When the underlying problems are not corrected, the heart may beat abnormally setting the stage for a potentially adverse event or worse , stop altogether. Life or death can be determined by the path of intervention chosen including emergent intervention such as CPR, defibrillation, and rescue medications.

In life there are often times when we are unaware that a problem exists. Children especially rely on us for proper care, treatment, and protection. Yet abuse occurs all around us. Providing victims with communication tools, an open non-judgmental environment, and trust are keys to survival. As parents we need to be aware of the needs of our loved ones, provide a solid foundation, and know when a particular event of behavior is not normal. It is imperative to act or intervene early on so that we may prevent further destruction of the individual or worse yet, death.

Way too often, our busy lives, or even denial, cloud our awareness of behavior changing events that could identify a treatable problem before it is too late. We need to be the rescuers of those in need. For me, in the long run, my heart literally and figuratively failed.

After mom died and things were being settled, Wally sent us away to Pennsylvania to stay with family for the summer; time he used to empty the house of my mother's belongings: literally empty. I'd like to believe that he was surrounded by loving friends as they divided her clothes, personal trinkets, and jewelry. I am convinced though that his friends were of the same character as he, leaving nothing behind for those rightfully entitled.

I began to develop a crush that summer of 1974, on a boy named Donny. He was my first "heart throb," but as luck would go, wanted little to do with me. I was freckle-faced, awkward, and probably way too desperate to be loved by him, go figure. He was the typical tall, dark, and handsome stereotype with a long, slender torso. He had a beautiful smile with perfect white teeth, incredible crystal blue eyes engulfed in long, thick black lashes. His demeanor was gentle and pleasantly kind. I was smitten; but my affection was not returned before we returned home. I felt dejected, this was the first relationship I would throw myself at despite not being wanted, and not the last. The summer went by quickly and soon we were back in to Buffalo!

A few summers later we returned to Pennsylvania with Carla, now married to Wally, and the whole family to visit Wally's relatives. I was now fourteen, still very infatuated with Donny and couldn't wait to see him again. I had become fully developed and was quite proud of who I had become (what he was missing out on).

As luck would have it he now took a liking to Roberta. I couldn't believe what was going on! I was disheartened and my ego took yet another blow. I could understand why Roberta was so attractive to young males. I guess she was "the whole package," sort of like Scarlett O'Hara that sat and waited while men swooned over her. She appeared to take pleasure in directing Donny's attention her way, knowing that I cared for him. I had practically thrown myself at him to get him to notice me. I had never experienced feelings of this intensity for anyone before. Those unfamiliar feelings coupled with my insecurity, and now jealousy; my emotions were bursting! Once again, I was rejected. I thought my feelings for Donny were love, but know now it was more likely curious lust and jealousy. I kept a journal that summer of my rampant emotions and raging hormones. In it I tried to understand myself, interpret my internal rumblings, and decipher if everything my heart was throbbing for was real. My journal was a place where I felt safe and could express each facet of what I was experiencing quite explicitly. I wanted him physically and had no limit to what I was willing to do for him.

In retrospect I shouldn't have wanted physical touch so desperately, especially from a boy who was rejecting me, but the need simply overwhelmed me! I wanted someone to love me, and me alone! His presence overcame my youthful senses. To this day I am proud to say that despite the insanity of all my needs, I didn't act on any of them in the end.

With each journal entry completed, I carefully placed the book in between my clothing in my suitcase where I could lock my secrets away–where my secrets would remain with me.

I guess it shouldn't have surprised me that somehow Wally and Carla came across the journal and read it. I remember that I was visiting at my Uncle Don's, Wally's brother, when the phone rang and it was for me.

"Hello?" I said inquisitively.

"I want you back here now!" The angry voice on the line was Wally and I knew not to argue. I ran all the way back to my Aunt Viola's, Wally's sister's house, to find the van packed. We left Pennsylvania abruptly, right then and there. I didn't know what was going on until I was scorned for my behavior in front of all my siblings, for having embarrassed them. There it was out in the open, my personal feelings, and my hatred for Roberta, and now guilt that it was my fault we left. I didn't know which emotion was more damaging: being mortified by them reading my diary, deeply violated, embarrassed, or being humiliated!

My diary was no longer packed in my suitcase: it was gone and I didn't dare ask for it back. I just didn't understand. Perhaps it was personal, perhaps intentional, I never knew. I just left to tuck my metaphoric tail between my legs. My first experience with love had been shredded, mutilated, and now dirty. It made me very confused.

Sometimes I wondered why I even continued to trudge forward. I felt my world should end and that I should blend into the background and disappear. Perhaps no one would notice.

The wounds healed, but I vowed then never to put my feelings in writing again. This was gravely unfortunate for me then because the one place I was safe, able to express myself, and process my feelings was through my writing. From then, and for a very long time forward, I turned everything inward developing a new pattern: failed relationships, lack of trust, and pushing people away.

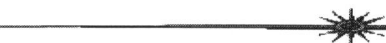

My first kiss was from a boy named John. He had dark brown hair, brown eyes, and glasses. He was very attentionate, attentive, athletic, intelligent, and had a deep calming voice. He was caring in many ways and I felt good around him. He came from a large family, deeply rooted in their faith. We had a lot in common but I was afraid I didn't know how to be in a real relationship. I broke up with him the next day because I was fearful of how I felt toward him and whether I could trust myself. I panicked because he cared for me and I didn't know how to accept it, nor felt I deserved it. I was probably more fearful of my family's reaction and the possibility of a horrific outcome.

Tommy was my first "spit swapping" boyfriend. He was less serious, which I liked. He also had dark features, but had a carefree twinkle in his eye. His stature was tall and slender, and his voice jovial. I had the same intimacy issues with Tom and when he kissed me I started to laugh. No, it wasn't funny, but I was unable to process the emotion. I broke up with him too.

From then on there were crushes, most of the boys that saw Roberta thought her to be beautiful but untouchable making me feel seconded and suspicious of their intentions. As a teenager, I didn't want to hear about Roberta anymore!

By ninth grade I had developed a body most guys lusted after. They were coming out of the woodwork to notice me! Everything about me was curvy, firm, and round including by full sized c-cup breasts! This created a whole new set of problems for me. I was getting a lot of attention for all the wrong reasons. As much as I was starving for attention I couldn't sort it out nor trust any of the boys liked me as a person. I just stopped taking interest in them because it was overwhelming and I was fearful of being hurt.

One day, my friend Karen came to me all excited. "Guess what? Ray Brophy wants to go out with you."

"Why?" I asked. "He doesn't know me."

"Well, he likes you and wants to know if you'll go jogging with him." I truly hated this game and didn't understand why he just didn't approach me himself.

"Point him out to me so I am sure who you are talking about," I told Karen.

I discovered he was a guy that I had once liked and thought was really cute, but believed to be out of my league and untouchable. I was pleasantly surprised but cautious knowing he had previously liked Roberta (*and she once liked him*). Now, he wanted to get to know me! I agreed to go jogging after school and was perplexed at his choice of activity. I was curious about him and somehow, it felt safe.

Ray was a shy football player with thick curly blonde hair, playful blue eyes, and a deep calming voice. I admit that jogging was out of character for me because I found it boring, it made me sweat, made my hair frizz, and my breasts bounced ridiculously. Modesty was something that I was still adjusting to. I asked him, "Why did you want to go jogging?"

"I thought you were a jock and it's the type of thing you would like to do," he replied.

In 1978 "jocks" were the athletic click and because I was a cheerleader it was guilt by association, although it wasn't true. I really didn't seem to fit in anywhere. I had no sense of commitment to anyone, however Ray would change that. We went to a movie on that Friday and he asked me to go "steady." I agreed thinking; *Maybe he will be different than the others.*

I found he was endearing and comfortable to be with, as well as an escape. He didn't publicly show affection, which made things so much more amicable. We stayed together throughout high school as the perfect couple; a cheerleader and football player, both captains of our teams.

We were like bookends, and he endearingly nicknamed me, "Bear."

After Ray and I started to become physically involved, we spent a great deal more time together experimenting. It was so natural: we were young and in love and neither had experience. Yet with him, I was eager to please and learned to love his touch.

We had the typical parental struggles; we couldn't kiss or do anything other than hold hands at my house. So we complied by taking long walks in the woods.

As we walked and talked endlessly, he would hold my hand the entire time, stopping only to hold me gently and kiss me.

As I became more and more comfortable with my physical self and exploring that side of me, I discovered that Wally and Carla were also taking a closer look. One day, Carla came into my bedroom to have a talk.

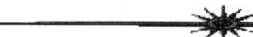

"Linda, we need to talk," she said. "It seems that you and Ray are getting a little too close and I worry that you may get pregnant," she continued.

I gave her credit for acting as a parent and approaching me about pregnancy and birth control, but to be honest I was insulted that she would think I would divulge that part of my life to her. She had never embraced me in that way and had not gained my trust; in fact there were times things that I had confided in her found their way back to me through Roberta. Talk about losing trust in someone. Of course I did what every paranoid teenager would. I denied it. "Ray and I are certainly not ready for that, I said with complete confidence."

I was indignant about needing her assistance let alone discussing sex!

Wally, on the other hand, developed a new behavior. He became very interested in me as a person. I found this rather odd, but as my self-esteem had grown with Ray, I thought maybe I had developed some "worth" to him. On Sundays, Carla would leave the house while I stayed home to prepare for the next week ironing clothes and washing laundry. At first Wally would startle me because he would be in the basement. He would engage me in conversation which made me uneasy.

"How are things going?" he would ask. At first I was taken off guard because I wasn't often with him one-on-one. As the weeks passed, Wally began to become more affectionate with me, putting his arm around me when he was talking, and sometimes playfully pushing me around. I had never experienced this attention from a parent and tried to gracefully accept it.

One Sunday the playfulness changed. He got more assertive and it became more of a test of strength with him. He grabbed my wrists and wouldn't let go and when I asked him to stop he seemed to enjoy that I was not enjoying this game. I'm sure he saw the panic in my eyes. I guess that was a "turn on" for him.

Until then I never noticed how sinister his laugh could be. He reached the point where he overpowered me and knocked me to the floor. I tried really hard not to let him see my fear.

"Please let me go," I pleaded, my voice trembling.

He proceeded to press his body upon mine, pinning me to the floor. As I looked up at his face I could not believe this was happening, he was finding pleasure in it. Never again did I ever iron my laundry on Sunday, or go into the basement alone, but he still sought me out.

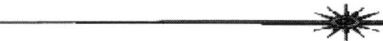

Ray never knew the dark secrets of my life. I feared he would desert me if I told him.

Reflection:

Forgiveness and acceptance are tools that I discovered were most significant to my survival at a young age. To forgive releases the negativity that keeps you in the past while accepting that understanding may never occur. My past is exactly that and by leaving it behind I am open to learn and grow. It took many years to forgive and it wasn't easy to come to this point. Yet, I was able to overcome many hurdles in order to love again, trust again, and live again. My life may not be perfect and there are times when I falter, but my experiences have given me the foundation I need to continue to survive.

I am grateful to have met Ray at such a young age. I was able to develop a healthy teenage relationship with him. It wasn't perfect, but it was a great beginning. As far as Wally, he violated the boundaries of trust between a parent and a child. It was his burden to bear and I have chosen to leave it behind. God has given me a wonderful ability to accept what I have no control over, and continue to move ahead.

If each man or woman could understand that every other human life is as full of sorrows, or joys, or base temptations, of heartaches and remorse as his own, how much kinder, how much gentler he would be.

William Allen White

A Self-Preserving Heart:

With each contraction of the heart approximately six liters of blood are transported through the entire cardiovascular system about three times per minute. This hollow muscular organ moves that blood through the circulatory system at a rate of 12,000 miles a day! Even more fascinating is the fact that it equates to about 500 miles per hour.

For most of us, our blood circulates about as fast as an airplane travels. In perspective this distance is equivalent to the drive between Buffalo and Boston. Ironically, Buffalo is where I live and Boston is where I chose to receive my heart transplant. The effectiveness of the heart as a muscle can be affected by many factors, just as traveling can be affected by road construction or traffic congestion. When a part of the body is not getting enough blood supply, the body can adjust to create collateral circulation, which allows blood flow and preventing that area from perishing. As a traveler, we may choose an alternate route, or even need to follow a detour. Simply put, survival occurs when we adapt to our surroundings rather than resist.

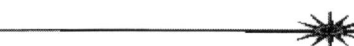

Each day I wake up and I am happy for that. If nothing heroic happened during the night, I slept well. So often my sleep was interrupted by overhead codes being called, helicopters coming in to the heliport, or ambulances racing through the streets. Often my thoughts turned to hope that, just maybe, the helicopter that woke me was bringing in a potential organ. That thought was somberly interrupted though when I realized that someone needed to die for that to occur. Someone's life will end tragically; someone's family will suffer so that I can survive.

Waiting for someone to die was a contradiction of my life and I thought it was selfish. I began to deeply reflect. I experienced this same scenario when my sister Patti needed a heart.

"How can I look toward survival as a positive thing when someone will die?" she would cry gasping for breath.

"Patti, if God's will is for you to live, then it will happen. God hasn't given man the technology in vain."

"I talked to a priest and even the church isn't clear on transplant. It's hard to accept it as what will save me if my God is not accepting." She was so deeply concerned.

I was ignorant then but seemed to have the right words to comfort her.

So, why do I doubt myself now? Well for one thing, it's different to put the shoe on the other foot, and possibly too because I am a nurse and my profession has been to save lives, not wish for lives to end. It is a struggle justifying what is right. *Why am I deserving of this gift?* I would think. *I should feel guilt, I should feel remorse.* This is what I told myself, yet inwardly I was excited about the possibility of my wait being over despite how it would occur. It seemed morbid.

On several occasions, I spoke in depth with Kristyn about the process of acceptance.

"It is not uncommon among transplant patients to feel the way you are feeling. In fact it is normal. What you need to realize is that they are your feelings and you are entitled to them."

Kristyn helped me recognize that there were two separate entities involved. Someone would not die for me to live.

"Someone will die, yes, but the end of his or her life was a separate entity, a separate book. As a result of that unfortunate event, you will be given a miraculous chance at life," she comforted me.

The nurses who took care of me also had a wonderful acceptance of how the process worked. To this day, I can't help but be grateful for the way their beautiful energy flowed into me as a patient. They shared numerous random acts of kindness such as brightening my days with little trinkets they purchased from the gift shop, cards they bought for me to send home to my family, and even treats from the nursing station. I especially enjoyed the security found from a furry stuffed animal and the comfort of chocolate. It is amazing to reflect on the simple pleasures you enjoyed looking into the eyes of your inner child. I learned to appreciate the difference between my wants and needs.

I needed nourishment, warmth, and a healthy outlook. I had it all here except love. So when people would ask what I needed I struggled to answer. Granted, hospital food isn't as good as home cooking, and the dress code entailed the standard blue gown and pants; the only thing I was truly missing was the immediate availability of my family. Reality was though that at any point or at any time I could access them through memories, by phone, through the internet, and if I had been more technologically prepared, I would have had my sky cam set up. Today's technology is amazing!

I also had my hospital family and often thought about how much we all shared despite the different paths we had come down to get to our present place. Our social group helped us express our inner torment to one another which helped us all see each other through. It was an interesting balance of good and bad days where we all seemed to take turns lifting one another up.

I was reminded on a daily basis that human nature in any crisis is to help, so when people did ask if I needed anything, instead of saying no, I would say, "I would love some Oreos, Pepperidge Farms cookies, or a Snicker's bar." As silly as it seems, accepting their offers of kindness helped on two levels. I had reminders that made me feel good when I was having a down moment, and those who brought the gifts felt good about bringing them. My friend Loren, from Jamaica Plains, a suburb of Boston, was one of my biggest fans! She made sure I had as many of life's indulgences as she could muster up when she visited. I especially enjoyed the "stuffed muffins" which we didn't have in Buffalo.

As the spring weather started rolling in, staff would comment about the weather improving. Danielle, my nurse stood at the window commenting, "You know, with more people being actively out in the community, there is more potential for available organs." She turned to me and smiled.

It was weird. Another morning one of the physician's rushed hurriedly into my room making rounds. "I drove recklessly to work this morning to find you a donor but had no luck," he jokingly said.

It took me a moment to connect to the hospital transplant humor and initially I thought it was a crazy thing to say. I am sure my facial expression proved my confusion. When I was able to mentally "connect the dots," and understand his sense of humor, it was actually quite funny.

It didn't end with the hospital staff though. My friend Tony and even Chris' cousin Mark made comments. "We are going to have to take matters into our own hands," they would tell me.

The implication was that they were going to make a few organs become available. I guess by going on an imaginary killing spree, it helped reduce their frustration and helplessness with my illness. I just knew they loved me.

One morning I asked Danielle, how she felt about the way loss of life impacted her patients, I found her reply quite fitting. She said, "I am here to take care of you. I know you, not them. I care about you getting well."

I was speechless and realized the reality of it. In general I was comforted.

A few days later, Danielle took me for a walk and allowed me to go outside to get some fresh air. She confided in me that her young cousin was in a car accident and it didn't look like she was going to make it. She continued talking, telling me the girl had problems with addiction and perhaps this was why she lost control of the car. I asked her to consider it an intervention from God and maybe it would be a path to a new beginning for her. As pained as Danielle was confiding her story, she confided that she hoped her family would be strong enough to donate the organs, because that was what helped save people like me. The girl passed away the next day. Her organs saved many.

I continued having my "senseless death dreams," especially after the subway train derailed in Boston. It was the first time in my life I had heard a "mass casualty code" called in a hospital. As a nurse I recognized it, feared the worst, hoped for the best. Similar to my dreams I'd prayed for the victims whose lives I could saved.

Now in my room over thirty days I began adapting to my role as a patient. For the first time in my life, I could be selfish and no one would judge. I didn't have anyone to take care of but me. I was there to get as healthy and rested as I could in preparation of the biggest event of my life. I needed to keep my stress level down, eat well, stay as active as I could, and grow in my faith. I now had an agenda.

I asked to see the physical therapist so that I could get started in an activity program. I needed to keep my muscles strong. I had already lost about ten pounds of muscle mass and was growing physically weaker.

Geoff, from my peer group, had been the next person to get his heart. Through the grapevine I heard that he had a difficult time.

Shield wrote on his Care page: "He is having trouble breathing and needed to be re-intubated."

The message sent a chill through our group. It would be several days and many interventions before Geoff was stable. Now, he was ready to go home. In his infinite wisdom this amazing man who had been through it all, encouraged me to stay strong. He stood at the foot of my bed before being discharged to go home delivering his message.

"Walk, as often as you can. I was so weak after surgery I couldn't stand. It is imperative for you to plan ahead," he told me.

Tearfully happy for him, yet sad to see him go, I got to work and asked for a physical therapy evaluation! Paul, the physical therapist, explained that there were a limited number of exercises that I could tolerate in order to maintain muscle and to prepare for my post-op recovery, but that the heart itself was at a point when any further physical stress would be unsafe. My cardiologist later explained that a sick heart uses much more energy to complete its basic tasks than a well heart uses. So I was at least blessed with a Pedi cycle and some exercise bands. I was told to pedal while watching television and rest during the commercials. I preferred pedaling during the commercials; it was exhausting! I worked with these as often as I could and "guilted" my hospital family peers to do the same.

I chuckled to myself thinking, *If the P.A. lines were portable, I could have started my own 'pedaling' class.*

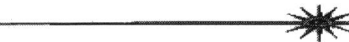

I asked to see the hospital chaplain, Katherine, so that she might help me gain spiritual strength. I needed to set things right in my life if I were to receive the gift of life and make things right with God. I met with her a few times a week. She would talk with me about biblical passages and give me readings to review after each visit. Sometimes I would feel panicked when I thought I may not have the right answers yet she never made me feel like my thoughts or perceptions were wrong. After meeting with Katherine and finishing the tasks I was assigned, I am happy to say that I made my First Holy Communion. That first experience of receiving host made everything worthwhile. I felt whole and my life enriched; definitely more complete. Katherine brought an incredible calm into my room when she was there and I welcomed it with open arms!

Another wonderful support for me was the young lady who volunteered her time to be the "book cart lady." She stopped in to visit every other week. On her cart were donated books as well as library books that you could sign out or even keep, if you chose. Her simple gesture of donating her time was often a lifesaver for me. I read everything I could get my hands on. I read the entire *Twilight* series that one of the nurses brought in for me. Someone even bought me the movie. I felt so connected! Everyone began to get involved in keeping me busy. Either that or they were concerned about what other things I was capable of after making Bessie and adopting Wilson! I received many movies to view, and CD's to listen to.

I even entertained Diva the hospitality dog, all of which helped me to brave the inevitable. I had continued to journal daily on my progress, but was cautious with this because my past experiences haunted me still.

As time passed, I became more familiar with some of the hospital equipment. In fact, there was a huge system of medical instrumentation in my room that I found intriguing, called the "boom." Just like on a sailboat, it was a large support pillar, but instead of sails, it was a hydraulic system with electrical power for vital intensive care level monitoring of all types. It was the epicenter of my room. I was well beyond any medical knowledge as a unit nurse and I was intrigued to learn all about it. I watched the nurses intently recognizing the tower could be moved without affecting the performance of equipment to optimize space, simply by pushing a button to release the hydraulics, and resetting it. Being the clever and resourceful girl that I am, I did just that. I created my own system and placement with the tower. By arranging my bed, hospital furniture, and adjusting the arms on the boom to certain positions, I could easily access my entire room and bathroom independently. That four foot leash was no longer a hindrance!

With my new freedom and my spirits lifted, I made the room more home-like, especially since Kenny and Lauren had already decorated theirs. I felt that old familiar competitive need to fit in coming to surface! I lined my movies up on a medicine cart, adding Wilson as the focal point for decoration. Cards were hung on the walls and bathroom door with medical tape. I positioned my flowers by color and arrangement so that they looked nice around the room. I also created bookshelves along the window sill. Each patient room was a good size allowing for couch beds, recliners and a sitting area for family members to stay. I set it up like a living room and decorated it to my taste.

It had been thirty-four days since I had seen Chris and he was finally well enough to visit. When he walked into my room, I have to admit it was like a fairy tale. I felt a rush of excitement as he hobbled toward me with the biggest nervous smile I had ever seen him wear. His clothes perfectly pressed, he was wearing a green pinstripe button down shirt that accentuated his green eyes. His shiny brown hair was slicked back, revealing his "widow's peak," and his glasses warmed his cheek and jaw lines. As I walked impatiently toward him, his excitement shone in his eyes, and I felt trembling in his touch. In his arms, while he held me, nothing else existed. To be deprived for so long of him physically, I thought I would explode. I was so overwhelmed with happiness I started to laugh! I know he was confused but laughing became something I did when an emotion was too intense to handle. I envisioned him being my "knight in shining armor," and didn't want to let go of that moment. I had waited so long to feel love of that intensity and I was so grateful to be able to experience it; unconditional, unsolicited love!

Vince peeked in from behind him. I was so grateful for his support. They brought me linens from home and some of my favorite foods. They even brought sponge candy for the nurses. Our visit went by too quickly. We spent what time we had together resting quietly in bed holding hands and sneaking off at times to pleasure one another. I embraced every moment with him.

Once Chris left, I made my bed with my own linens from home. Chris brought a great multi-colored comforter set complete with curtains and throw pillows. I coerced my nurse, Karen to help me to hang the curtains! They all learned how creative I could be with simple hospital supplies. Some basic tape along the top edges of the curtain valance and some carefully tied knots in the fabric created a decorative home away from home. It wasn't perfect, but it was quite comfortable.

I learned to appreciate every act of kindness; phone calls, e-mails, and gifts simply recognizing how much I was loved by so many dedicated friends, family, and medical staff.

Loren also continued to visit. We had worked together in Buffalo and somehow we managed to reconnect by e-mail before I ended up in Boston. She had a brand-new baby with her partner Sara and parenting had become quite the eye-opener for them both. When I was in the hospital, Loren would pop in spreading her positive energy and warmth everywhere. We'd get so caught up in conversation that we'd lose track of time. She would visit armed with "goodies" to enjoy. I developed a two-cookie limit, mainly to keep myself from over indulging, but also so that I could entice the nurses to come in to visit me more often. I enjoyed reading the books she brought and especially enjoyed the *Ally McBeal* CD collection when I needed to be mindless and simply laugh. What a wonderful bonus from a beautiful friend!

With each admission to the hospital, Dr. Seideman and Barbara would check in on me from the lab offering gentle words of wisdom and kindness. They were like guardian angels who never failed to go way above and beyond for me. From moral support to nail polish, they supported me to the best of their abilities while remaining conscientious of the boundaries separating hospital care and the genetics lab: separate entities. They communicated through the hospital team and I was fortunate their studies were at a point that they needed follow-up with my children. As a result, my children were brought to Boston for a few days to assist with the study and spend some vital time with me, just before Easter. So many pieces of my life came together through the kindness and generosity of others. Some days, while in the middle of some of my darkest moments, those angels lifted me to cloud nine. Scott was discharged on Easter Sunday which made the day exceptionally special.

Reflection:

They say we often can't see the forest through the trees. I don't know where that saying came from but it is so true. Life can be great or it can be devastating but at the end of every life experience there is a lesson. At the time we are experiencing a difficult or even a joyous time, it is so important not to become so consumed in the moment that we forget to notice the little things, the precious things, the beautiful things that fill our hearts..

Everyday I spent in the hospital; I was blessed with a new lesson, or a better understanding of myself. Instead or remaining guilt riddled knowing that my children were inflicted with my genetic blueprints, I am sure that I wouldn't have done anything differently in my life. I love my children more than my own life, and see the medical advancements in technology that can save them. I was able to take advantage of an opportunity for survival so that I could be here to support their own individual journeys. This is my "silver lining."

POTHOLES

Each day has the potential to start with a sunrise and end with a sunset. I read once that a sunset is God's final portrait of the day. While I was in the hospital I made it a part of every single day to marvel at what I would call His photo album.

"When circumstances seem impossible, when all signs of grace in you seem at their lowest ebb, when temptation is fiercest, when love and joy and hope seem well-nigh extinguished in your heart, then rest without feeling and without emotion, in the Father's faithfulness."

-Daniel Tryon

Chapter 7

A Cold Heart: Numb to Emotion

They say that the heart is an organ of passion and strong emotion. When you are happy you can feel the excitement in your chest and with each increased heart beat you may feel it flutter. When you are sad or disappointed your heart can be said to be broken and it can feel heavy and flaccid like a water balloon, stunned, or numb. Left unprotected emotional heartache will lead to physical heartbreak.

Throughout my life, my heart lacked emotion and I shielded myself from knowing its existence. The usual physiological and innate or learned response to external stimuli became flattened, enabling me to move forward, unyielding to my surroundings.

The heart is believed to be an organ of divine attributes or truth. Whether it is spiritual, emotional, moral, or intellectual, it is amazing how much can be attributed to this hollow muscular organ that is no larger than your fist.

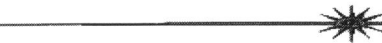

Some people look at a shamrock plant and think of the trinity as it has three leaves on one branch. When I look upon this plant, I think of my sisters, our connection, and the love the three of us had. We were one family, one unit with an everlasting love. Some people say that I am responsible for severing a limb of the plant, by choosing to end my sister's life: allowing my sister's death. Truthfully, nobody should ever have to be put in a place where he or she needs to determine if a loved one lives or dies. It is another pain that will haunt me forever. Yet, I know emphatically that I made the correct choice.

As a child, I remember that Patti was independent and had her own methods of surviving. She carried her wounds as badges. Her mood was unpredictable and it was difficult to get truly close to her. The fact that she was my half-sister didn't matter to Joyce and me. As far as we were concerned, she was the big sister. My dad loved her as his daughter. Despite her legal place in our home, Patti seemed to lack connection and seemed emotionally empty.

She knew little about her father other than he didn't want a daughter, he rejected her. I always felt Patti wanted the chance to show her biological father who she became thinking he would love her now. I think this became an even greater need when she fell ill. We all wanted the same things, grasping for it anyway we could.

Patti was able to love, but I believe she feared getting close. She was fortunate as she created her own haven away from our home for most of her formative years. She would spend as much time as possible with her best friend Terry, becoming part of her family for over twenty-seven years. They lived on the hill about one-quarter mile away and Patti was thrilled with the unofficial adoption.

She seemed to find solace in their home. The Metzgers were an exuberant family with eight children. They loved life, laughter, and especially music. Their family was very faith-based and created a wonderful environment for Patti's lonely, broken soul. She was there every day after school, soaking in the normalcy of everyday life with a solid family. I have to be honest, I envied her for that. I was angry that she did not take us with her. Later I met Karen.

Patti had grown into a beautiful young woman with clear, delicate skin, and serene blue eyes. She wore glasses that hid the rounded features of her beautiful face. I would laugh when she took them off because she would need to press on the sides of her eyes to clear her vision, distorting her face to focus, rather than just put them back on. It seemed silly, but I wondered if she deliberately tried to appear unattractive.

She dressed in Puritan, flowing clothes, perhaps so that Wally would not notice her hourglass figure. Yet, all the years with the abundant love of the Metzgers could not disguise the anger within her. Her radiant face carried that trace of hostility.

My sister Patti was tough to get along with. In fact, sometimes she was downright mean! Sometimes I was thrilled if she talked to me, while at other times I knew to stay clear for fear she would strike out. She seemed to need to maintain a threatening presence in our home, which was contradictory to the way she portrayed herself through her musical talent.

She could play any instrument harmoniously–enveloping you unexpectedly. Admittedly, it was rough in the beginning when her first instrumental choice was the clarinet, but I grew to love that instrument's melodic trance. She became one with her instruments, peaceful and calm, whether the trumpet, drums, or piano. It was as if the world was on hold as she performed. I wonder now if she is playing in Heaven

As Patti grew older she increasingly resembled my mother. Her hair darkened and grew long and wavy. She had mom's contagious laugh. Back then, we didn't have large barreled curling irons, so we would use orange juice cans as rollers to straighten the kinky, curly look or if we had less time, using a regular clothing iron would do. Our curly hair demanded maintenance if we didn't want to look like Medusa, and because of this Patti rarely wore her hair down. I became increasingly comfortable with her hair pulled tightly in a more militant bun.

Although adult support lacked, it was my sister Patti who taught me the facts of life shortly after my mom passed. She took on the role of the mother figure when she was thirteen and came forward with the "truth," while I was sleeping in my bunk bed. She sat on the edge of my bed, woke me up, held up a book and allowed me to settle in the corner of the bed for my first lesson. My sister gave me a black and white marbled notebook and a pen. "Here are some terms you need to know," she said. "Spell fallopian tube."

There I was with my pink sleeping bag curled up around me and a bewildered face.

"Go on, put it down," she demanded, then added, "I'll say it again, fal-lop-i-an tube," Enunciating it very slowly.

There she sat, Patti with her long, curly, brown hair pulled tightly back into a ponytail. She had distant blue eyes hidden by her glasses, high cheekbones and a smile just like my mother's. Patti was very sensitive to the gap between her front teeth and the cleft in her chin, but she could be volatile so we knew not to tease her about it.

I was a little shy of this "life lesson," probably a little immature to be receiving it from her at nine-years-old. I could feel my cheeks becoming flushed from embarrassment as my lesson made me feel trapped. I was just barely ten at the time. It was one more time in my life I felt very uncertain, insecure and once again missed my mother. The lesson continued until I knew the correct terminology of all the reproductive parts of the male and female anatomy as well as what they were used for. Although somewhat embarrassing, it was necessary. Perhaps this was the beginning of my nursing career. Void were the times of endearment shared between mother and daughter, the exchange of thoughts, values and lessons in life. Patty gave to me what she knew, the same lesson that was being taught to her at school.

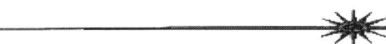

At 17-years-old, she left our home and enlisted in the Army, leaving Joyce and I behind. I wanted her to stay, wanting desperately not to be left alone with Wally, but I knew she had to find her own way, as did Joyce and I. She was no longer just a quarter mile down the road. When she closed the door to our house, somehow the door to sexual abuse for me also closed. We never talked about it, but I was silently grateful to her for somehow putting an end to something that should never have started. Still to this day, I am not sure what role she played or how she was able to end it; perhaps she threatened to tell the world the truth. The only thing that mattered is she helped me before she left, because that is what sisters do.

Shortly after her departure, she married Steve. My family was certain to blame me for some sort of awareness or involvement. Once again, I was playing defense for my sister. Instinctively I fought for her, even if I did not know what I was fighting for. Somehow the situation made me feel we were back together as a team, even with her physical absence. I became the focal point of the negativity surrounding her actions, but I felt her strong and positive in spirit. I wondered why my step-parents burdened me with this perceived game versus acting as responsible adults and addressing her personally. Once again it appeared the roles were confused.

"You must know something, she writes to you! Who is this man she married? Was she pregnant? What color is he?" they badgered me.

My family was certain that I knew something about the details of her abrupt marriage and pressed me relentlessly for the details. I wondered why any of it really mattered.

I wrote her a letter explaining the inquisition that I was going through. I explained to her that it was wearing me down and I was doing everything I could to preserve her dignity. I pleaded with her to contact Wally and Carla to make things right so we could all move on. I couldn't stand the degradation; like pointed guns as she stood blind sighted. In my mind she was just dealing with her own issues of loneliness and abandonment marrying a man whose first words to her were, "Hey you've got a zit!"

Terms of endearment were not a trademark for Patti, but when I mailed her the letter, she was quick to respond, complete with a picture, confirming his ethnicity. A year later, she did not need to send pictures; she was coming home with her new baby, Shawn.

He was a little sweetheart! He had bright blue eyes that twinkled when he smiled, and his mom's thick brown hair. Shawn had a cleft in his chin, just like my sister, and looked a lot like her.

It concerned me that Patti had become so heavy from the pregnancy, and how often she and Steve went out to eat fast food. The Patti I once knew had been weight conscious, slender, and an accomplished cross-country runner in New York State. I wondered what part of her changed allowing herself to fall apart. I noted PattI's feisty energy was gone.

With this first real exposure to Steve, Patti and her family stayed with us for a short period of time. Carla obtained a crib for Shawn and placed it in my room for them to stay, allowing them privacy. I slept on a couch bed we kept in the hallway adjacent to my room. It was my first true experience with exhaustion, lack of sleep, and the demands of parenting. Shawn had demands both day and night! Patti seemed to be the one tending to his needs ensuring he didn't disturb his father.

Her new husband appeared to have two distinct personalities. At first he was probably the one she fell in love with; the polite military man full of charm and wit. The other was an abrasive, opinionated, aloof man. I tried to like him, really I did. Yet, I could see all the negative changes in my sister and felt his presence in her life played a role in these changes. She appeared afraid of him.

She was no longer the independent, self-motivated woman of stamina I once knew. My sister the marathon runner, whose eyes once hailed victory, now read defeat. My sister was replaced with a lethargic presence that lacked spark and didn't even seem to have enough energy to run to the refrigerator anymore! She had cut her hair short in a wash and go curly style. She no longer wore make-up, and dressed in tent-like maternity clothes. Her flat affect and dazed awareness disguised the beauty that was once so apparent. Her only predictability was her response to her child and to Steve's demands. Slowly, she appeared to be falling apart.

Steve treated her poorly and talked down to her in front of us most of the time. Initially we anticipated a brawl, like we would have endured if one of us had treated her that way, yet instead, she was complacent. He placed unrealistic demands on her and she dubiously met them. He was inconsiderate and would abruptly leave the house without explanation. It was very difficult to live with Steve. He was selfish, taking care of only himself, did not clean up after himself, and left reminders of his presence everywhere he went including his dirty laundry and dishes. When their family finally left, I was relieved. I knew that I would miss my sister, but it was also painful to be in her presence knowing that she was only the shell of the person I knew and loved.

A Cold Heart: Numb to Emotion

A few years later, Patti got pregnant with my niece, Cassie. By then, I was married and had a home of my own. They had now moved to Minnesota, away from my family, and near Steve's. My sister remained in the Army there and we didn't speak very often. I got to know her daughter Cassie through pictures only. Her appearance was a combination of her dad and my sister. She had his narrow blue eyes and sharp chin, but curly, lighter brown hair. After delivering Cassie, Patti told us that the doctor informed her, "Something is wrong with your heart." It wasn't long after that Patti returned to Buffalo and was placed on a heart transplant list at our Veterans hospital. It was 1985 and the hospital was newly accredited for transplant surgery.

It was with the second pregnancy that gave her heart away, literally, and I believe in spirit as well. It was in the hospital where Patti would remain to wait for her new heart. Patti would be the second in our family, second to my cousin Sharon in 1979.

Steve on the other hand lived with Carla and Wally until he overstayed his welcome.

Despite the extenuating circumstances involving his wife and family, Steve never wavered from old habits. The children were often left behind while he went out carousing the town for endless hours, lying about his whereabouts. Patti would call looking for him and no one had answers. Wally and Carla just tried to protect her feelings by not unveiling their frustration or the truth. Eventually, Steve was asked to leave and went to the Ronald Mc Donald home.

Patti remained in the hospital for over two months during which time she never wavered in her support of him.

We weren't privy to her disappointment for the lack of support Steve continuously demonstrated. Their relationship spiraled downhill, especially when Patti learned that the Ronald McDonald House was even having difficulty with his long absences. Steve had been thoughtlessly leaving the kids behind, not recognizing their need for food and diapers. There, Steve continued to use Patti's illness to lure people in to assisting him. He took advantage of their compassion and understanding in a difficult situation.

After the transplant Patti secured the best possible life and home she could with her family. She rented a home in a small town called Derby, just outside of Buffalo, and planned to make things work with her marriage to Steve. At this point they had survived solely on her disability while Steve searched for a job. Patti became a different person after her surgery. She was kind and generous with a gentle caring, nature. She became involved in the church and raising her family. She was loved by so many people and I got to know her on a much a different level. She believed God would provide for her and continued to endure. The surgery had changed her and God became the center of her life.

Her needs were simple, clothes for the kids, basic supplies, and a safety net. Steve felt the kids didn't need anything including gifts to celebrate birthdays and holidays. It made me uncomfortable and I could sense the disappointment in her demeanor when she would tell us, "We are celebrating Shawn's birthday as a family this year." "Steve doesn't want gifts or cake," she said to me holding back tears.

To compensate, we utilized church events to obtain some necessities including basic clothing, and food staple items. She had developed many friends both inside and outside the congregation.

Steve didn't like the kids to be present when he was watching television; especially football. He was an avid Buffalo Bills fan. He would send them to their rooms for hours at a time, and when he yelled in that house the "earth shook!" It wasn't uncommon to find the kids with their doors closed.

During these times we would all take refuge escaping for a walk or going to my home for the day. It would be there the kids could play as the children they were and we could be sisters.

My sister Joyce and I visited as often as we could and tried to ignore the uncomfortable circumstances. On rare occasions Patti would slip and tell the truth about his failure to support the family, about his militant ways, and rigid parenting. I didn't understand her bowing down to him; especially since she outranked him in the military. My suspicion confirmed: she was very afraid of him, but not nearly as afraid as she was of being alone. It was stressful for me to hear of all the stories, and I didn't understand her choice to remain in a bad situation after being blessed with the gift of life: a new beginning. She saw it more as an end for hopes of anything more. She believed in her commitment to marriage before God.

We compensated spending all the time we possibly could together again sharing our lives, becoming the sisters we were meant to be. Absent from Steve, her spunk returned, and she glowed. I thanked God for the opportunity to get to know her this way, that I was afforded this opportunity despite it only being a few short years. She was my sister, and my friend.

Some days our lives were carefree and wonderful like a movie you would see on the "Hallmark Channel." We would work out to videos and to this day as we "huffed and puffed" doing aerobics, I can hear her talking.

"You know, your head weighs about thirteen pounds," the instructor would state.

"Well then cut it off!" she would remark sarcastically.

Afterward we would reward ourselves with ice cream sundaes. We would load all the kids in wagons and strollers and go to the park, the beach, or anywhere we could escape the rigid realities of life. Inside her "wall of acceptance for the present" was a little girl who wanted to be valued and loved. It broke my heart not only for her, but all three of us girls, having fallen into bad relationships. We would talk for hours sipping herbal tea snuggled on the porch; unspoken words of disappointment loomed in the air. Such fortunate memories will forever remain in a very special place in my heart.

As we grew together, Steve fell apart. He tried a few jobs, but failed. He took an interest in photography and decided this was his new career. They lived on a wing and a prayer with Patti continuing to finance his dreams. She purchased all the necessary equipment and even helped him to create a studio in their garage. I will admit he did take nice pictures, if you were fortunate enough to receive them. Often he took the money for himself–leaving my sister to pay the debt. I felt the man had no soul.

When Steve and my sister were together, gone was the fun-loving, pillar of strength I grew to love and back was the meek, passive stranger. There were many teary days where I wanted her to go out on her own, but she had given up on love. She had accepted this lifestyle as all she would ever have.

"My only prayer is that I will live long enough for my kids to remember me. If I am ever in a situation where I am given a choice to do this again, receive a heart I mean, to save my life, I would not do it again," Patti somberly told me.

I was saddened but believed that her gift of life had afforded us a world of opportunity as sisters. Yet I could see, she had no self-esteem, no self-worth, and saw little to live for. It was painful knowing her despair, seeing the pain in her weary eyes, and the tears in her smile.

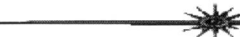

One day the phone rang and Patti was on the other end simply hysterical. "Steve slit his wrists and locked himself in the bathroom!" Patti cried.

Silently I wished he had been successful: at something. It could've been so much easier then and my sister could have had her life back. I felt guilty for feeling this way and prayed about it, yet felt somehow justified; he had somehow robbed my sister of her life.

"Did you call an ambulance?" I asked.

"Yes, it's on the way; I just don't want to be here alone," Patti continued.

"Where are the kids?" I asked.

"I am not sure, I think they ran to their rooms when they saw the blood," she told me.

"Are you alright?" I asked.

"I will be better once you are here, please come," she said.

"I'll be right over," I said as I hung up the phone.

When I got there, the ambulance was leaving and my sister Patti followed behind with Joyce agreeing to drive. Joyce had witnessed the entire event and they furiously cleaned up the blood before I got there. I found Cassie and Shawn hiding in their rooms and took them home.

In the hospital, Patti was approached by the doctor. "Steve's attempt on his life was not life-threatening because fortunately he sliced his wrists horizontally, not vertically. The blood loss was minimal. We have a psychiatrist evaluating him to determine if it is safe to return him home."

The incident was blamed on an "overuse" of nasal spray medication and Steve was released from the hospital. Once recovered, he decided that he needed the structure of the Army, and with or without Patti; he was re-enlisting in the Army. Of course, she was "with him."

They ended up moving from Buffalo to North Carolina as she bravely chose to support her husband and keep her family together. Us "Three Musketeers" would once again be separated. We were all fearful that Patti wasn't strong enough to endure it alone; more so, would be too far away from her medical providers: always trust your gut.

A Cold Heart: Numb to Emotion

A few months later, in the fall of 1990, I received a call in the middle of the night; it was Patti. There was an incredible rumbling sound in the background. She was almost unintelligible.

"What is that awful noise?" I asked.

"It's the plane engines, but I can't tell you more than that," she told me. "I just wanted to let you know that you may not hear from me for a few days, and not to worry," she continued.

I knew this was a military event and that due to confidentiality reasons, I couldn't ask any questions. It would only be a short time before the media would announce the truth; Steve was sent to the Gulf War.

"Are you coming home?" I asked.

"No, Steve wants me to stay here in our home." Her voice was complacent; almost disappointed. Again I was concerned for her, being so far away left to raising the kids – now without any support.

Those concerns didn't quiet and I was thrilled when my sister Joyce announced she was going to North Carolina to be with Patti. Joyce arrived only to validate our fears. Patti had taken ill but adamantly refused to come back to Buffalo.

"It's just a cold and Steve says he's sick of everyone treating me as if I am not normal," Patti argued.

The point was, she *wasn't* normal; she had a heart transplant and needed to always take extra precautions! Against everyone's wishes and Joyce's chagrin, Patti decided she was going to ride it out. Two days later, Patti was emergency flown back to Buffalo in cardiac distress, with Joyce and the children trembling beside her. As Patti was rushed to the hospital, I met Joyce and the kids at the airport. My poor Joyce began to fall apart.

"It was awful," Joyce sobbed now melting into my shoulder. "I am afraid she is going to die." All went silent as we finished the drive.

With Steve at war in the Gulf, CNN was attempting to locate him so that he could be flown home. I never saw my sister alive again, but spoke to her briefly when she was admitted to the hospital. Patti always had a way of minimizing the severity of a situation in order to protect us. I assured her that the kids would stay with me now, and that they would be O.K. Joyce remained traumatized.

"How are you doing?" I asked

"I'm alright," Patti's voice was weak. "They think its rejection, so they want to try a new medication," she continued barely getting the words out.

"How do you fell about it?" I asked.

"I'm tired of being sick, I'll do what I need too," she replied and the phone grew silent. Her social worker, Michelle, finished the call saying Patti was tired and needed to rest.

I never spoke to my sister again, but instead I heard from Michelle.

"You will all need to come to the hospital, things don't look good," Michelle said somberly.

When we all arrived, we were greeted by Michelle and the E.R. doctor.

"She has been placed on life-support. Her heart wasn't strong enough to endure the OKT3 medication. We attempted to revive her twice but her heart had stopped for ten minutes the first time and fifteen before we ended the code. That is a long time for the brain not to be perfuse properly. We are unsure what level of damage there is to the brain, but the heart is badly damaged. If there is brain activity, the only hope for survival would be another transplant." *The medication called OKT3 should have eradicated the massive rejection to save her life, but instead took it,* I thought to myself. Then it hit me. Memories of her wishes haunted me, entrenched deep in my mind, not wanting to be recanted. I feared I wasn't strong enough to honor her wishes.

Fortunately, the decision became blatantly clear and easy. Patti had been declared brain dead. We were now faced with the most tragic of decisions. "There is nothing left to be done," they said, "we need permission to remove the life-support: to 'pull the plug'."

It is a sad blur. My heart broke for Joyce who rode home on that plane where Patti begged for help. There was nothing any of us could do. I will never forget my last phone conversation with Patti, or how brave and accepting she was. I knew in my heart what needed to be done. Steve was back from the war now in time to legally make decisions.

"Let her go," I whispered. Steve looked at me nodding.

"No!" cried Roberta, "you are killing her. You can't give up; you have to give her a chance."

Steve made the final decision; the right decision, to let Patti go.

Despite heavy scrutiny from the rest of the family, we prepared for the procedure to end her life, each allowed to privately say our goodbyes. I cried beside her bed. I talked to her, feeling the most defeated I could ever recall. "I am doing what you asked of me, the toughest decision I have ever been involved in," I told her.

As I prayed, I watched a tear roll down her cheek. When there was no more time left, I kissed her and said goodbye. I joined my family in the hall where we stood peering into the glass walls of her room. When the ventilator was removed, of course we hoped she would take that breath. It was not the case as we were frozen in that moment.

Afterward, Roberta turned on me. "You killed her!" she cried, "this shouldn't be how she died." She continued screaming directly at me.

Anger welled up in me against the family that had always judged me and made me feel inadequate. I felt that they never knew my sister the way I did, nor did they know her wishes. I was an adult now and refused to be converted to that insecure child fighting for what was right. It wasn't long after that I chose to no longer associate with my "step-family."

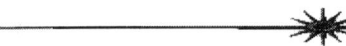

The wake was unbearable and gut-wrenching. Cassie, Patti's 8-year-old daughter walked in holding hands with my daughter Amanda who was seven. They had a wonderful bond and were truly connected. Upon seeing the casket, Cassie buckled at the knees and began to wail hysterically.

"Noooooo! She's not dead!" Her cries echoed above all tears and conversation and were heard throughout the funeral parlor. There wasn't a dry eye around and almost everyone began to sob.

For me, I was sent back in time to my mother's funeral reliving Aunt Rita's devastation. I was paralyzed in the moment as a pattern of recreated tragic memories was thrust upon us.

Amanda wrapped Cassie in her arms and together they lost control. "Mom," she would later tell me, "I needed to protect Cassie." "I needed to be brave," she continued.

I believe this may have been the beginning of Post Traumatic Stress Disorder (PTSD) for the two of them. Shawn took it all in, a brave little soldier, saying very little. I often wondered if this was part of the militant upbringing or if he truly understood it was mom's time. They were very close.

The funeral itself was done with complete military respect. The American flag was draped over her casket. The music and readings were done by the Metzger family, her true family, and the service ended with "Taps" somberly being played on the bugle. It was a wonderful tribute to my sister, my friend, a military leader, and wonderful mother.

Putting life together afterward was difficult. Steve adamantly wanted to return to war, leaving the kids with me. He just couldn't accept his loss and wanted to run. He wanted nothing to do with staying in Buffalo and its terrible memories.

"Buffalo is a terrible place with painful memories. I can't be here alone to raise these kids," he ranted.

I couldn't comprehend any of it, yet reminded him that those kids had just lost their mother and did not need to lose him too. I still believed in keeping family together, recalling the pain I felt when my mom died and feeling rejected by family.

Ray and I opened our home to Steve and the children after much debate. I reached out to this man despite how much he hurt my sister and how much I blamed him for her demise. Despite how I felt about Steve, my sister's family ultimately stayed in my home.

After all that we had been through, Steve continued all his inconsiderate habits and behaviors. There he had a birds-eye view of my weakened relationship with my husband Ray. He preyed on that.

I couldn't grieve Patti's death because I was overwhelmed with responsibility and lack of support. With five children under the age of eleven, there was little time to breathe. On top of that I had two men, a husband and brother-in-law, who were frequently nowhere to be found.

Day-after-day, Steve would just take off, spending insurance money anyway he could. He compensated for his absences by bearing gifts for me.

"Thank you for taking care of my kids," he told me.

I would rather have food on the table or clothes on the kids' backs. I accepted with reluctance and tried to be gracious thinking that it was his way of coping. Rarely did he buy for the kids.

One Saturday we took the kids out for a ride in the van. "Hey Steve, let's stop at Carvel for ice cream." He pulled in and parked. Steve got out of the car and returned with a single cone for me and nothing for the children. I was beside myself and couldn't bring myself to eat it. I choked back tears offering it to them and the six of us shared it.

"I bought that for you," he scowled, "kids quit begging."

All I could think as I snuck bites to the kids was, *This is how my sister lived.*

There were days that I was defeated by it all. One Saturday in November of that year, I was just plain exhausted and went back to bed while the kids watched television. I needed to cry and to be alone. Upon Steve returning from one of his road trips, he came in to check on me. He began to rub my back and for a brief moment I thought he was not such a bad guy: that was until his hands wandered into the rubber band of my panties. I abruptly stopped him flashing back to my childhood in horror! I fought to compose myself, telling him, "I am not interested in you that way." "Yes, I miss my sister and I am weary, but I have a husband and children," I cried.

He somehow interpreted my weakened relationship with Ray as an opportunity for "us" as a couple.

"Let's face it," he began, "it is obvious you and Ray are not happy." "You are a wonderful mother to all the kids. They get along well together. I am lonely and want a wife.

The kids need a mother. It is perfectly obvious what we should do," he finished.

It slapped me in the face. He believed that we were supposed to be a family and raise the kids together. Instantaneously, I was thrust into a flashback of my Aunt Joanne's death, my mom marrying my uncle after her sister's death. It was like a bad movie and I was numb!

Perhaps my mistake was the interpretation of the gifts he gave me or maybe, just like when I was a child, I was supposed to be somehow thankful to him for something. I was greatly confused and stunned. I wished it made sense.

I never told Ray what happened and Steve seemed to be humiliated. After that I rarely saw him, and the kids and I went on with our lives. From that point, I learned he had begun to date a woman who I had gone to high school with. He "wined and dined" her every night and rarely came home to the kids. It was very frustrating! In December, just three months after my sister passed away Steve announced he was getting married to Sunny.

My protective bubble surrounded me dulling my shock. Inside my heart cried for my sister. She deserved a little more respect than this, yet I reminded myself that this was Steve's style. Women mourn, men move on. I denied him and he moved to Sunny. I had learned more about men in my twenty-five years than I cared to know. I had two men in my home both absent in emotion and filled with selfishness.

Ray lacked interest, content with life as it was and saw things as fine. Steve was filled with ego and saw it as an opportunity for people to serve him as he had served his country. He lacked common sense; he was oblivious to social skills, political correctness, morals, and ethics. To him I was an opportunity!

My only goal was trying to care for the kids and keep my pants on! His was to get married and leave the kids with me so that he and Sunny could adjust to getting to know one another. Again I was flabbergasted that I existed in such a backward world! My response was, "Absolutely not!" For the first time in my life I developed a backbone. I told him his new life with his new wife was to begin as a family and that included his children.

My heart was broken seeing them prepare to go. I wanted to cling to my sister through them. I have no idea what he told the children all these years, about me, about "us," why they moved out, yet I wouldn't have permission to ask. Though I am certain, that none of it favorably reflects me.

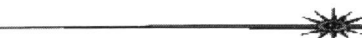

On the day of the wedding, I felt compelled to open a door to Sunny and offer her some support. I placed a call to her home. "Sunny, I have known you a long time and have a great deal of respect for you. Yet by marrying Steve, you become the step-mother of two of the most important people in my life: Shawn and Cassie. I am entrusting you with their care.

"As for Steve, I am not sure what he has told you but there is not any 'love lost between us.' In fact I have concerns for your well-being. I wish you well in your lives together. I know Steve's history. Keep your eyes wide-open, protect yourself, and mostly take care of my niece and nephew."

She thanked me and assured me she would. Sunny was a wonderful mother to the kids and created a life for them which included my family. I am grateful to her for her role in their lives; saddened I didn't play a more active role.

It was as if history was repeating itself when this initiated and I felt like I had abandoned my niece and nephew like I felt my Aunt Rita had done to us so long ago. I had been too young to understand. It was a difficult cross to bear, but they had a father and I didn't want to be a part of breaking up the biological family they had. I have never been confident whether I had made the right decision or not.

Years later, Sunny invited me to attend Shawn's college graduation. She and Steve were going through a divorce and she asked for my company. We rode together and I listened intently as she talked.

"You were right about Steve. Our entire marriage was full of lies and manipulation: every gift, every card, and every bouquet represented a fallacy."

"I am sorry to hear that, I hoped he had changed," I comforted her.

I was saddened that he continued to struggle to learn how to love despite being blessed with two wonderful, supportive wives. Listening to her, I saw the commitment and passion she had for my niece and nephew, raising them as her own. I couldn't have been happier as I was listening to her, validating I had made the right decision entrusting her to raise my niece and nephew.

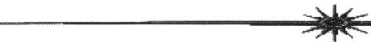

My sister would've been proud of her son when he walked across the stage as a St. Bonaventure University graduate, served the United States Army in Iraq, then walked down the aisle to marry his college sweetheart Meghan.

When I became sick, his communication with me grew very quiet. I sensed his fear and remembered his pattern of isolating himself when he worried. I picked up the phone to talk to Shawn about the way he may be feeling. He validated his fear that history might repeat itself. We had a wonderful conversation and I fell in love with the man he had become. He wanted to start a family but was afraid. I am happy to report that just eight months after my transplant, Shawn learned he didn't contract this gene and was expecting his first baby with Meghan!

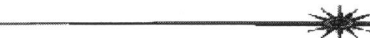

Cassie married and gave birth to a son, Braden. Unfortunately she fell victim to drug and alcohol abuse. As a teenager, she was a "cutter" and had many self-esteem issues as well as suffering from depression. For a while, when Cassie was on medication her happiness was outwardly overdone. She lacked the ability to appropriately express sadness and was unable to cry. I tried to intervene, tried to fill the void where her mother once existed. It was never enough.

Her son was diagnosed with a congenital heart problem and Cassie called me in hopes of disconfirming the family heart disease. I was able to remind her that since she didn't have the gene, her son could not be affected. Her continued inner turmoil led to her divorce, plus she lost custody of her son. I believed at that time, it was the best possible solution so that she could regain control of her life. It is not the case.

Occasionally Cassie will reach out to me. I regret not always being as compassionate as she needed me to be when she would ask me as an adult to, "Tell me about my mother." I wished I had taken a more loving role with Cassie and told stories of her beautiful mother, reminding her of the roots she came from, but sometimes I felt she should've known. Before my sister died, her wishes were that she lived long enough that they remembered her. Psychologically, I knew she held on for as long as she could, and I couldn't bear the thought that her kids lacked a solid memory of her. I wanted my sisters wishes validated, yet neglected to remember how the traumatic events may have impacted them. I failed to recognize Cassie's desperate grasp for a lifeline.

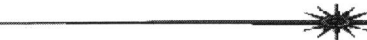

Years later, fast forward to today, Steve again did remarry and I assume he is happy, but I wonder about his new wife. Did the pattern continue? Was she another victim of his psychological abuse and web of lies or was God gracious enough to help him to grow?

I learned that he has health issues and I pray for his healing and recovery. It's not my place to ask any questions. That chapter of my life ended a long time ago but I am proud to know that his children stood by his side. They were raised well.

Reflection:

It is ironic where the twists and turns in life lead us, and the lessons that can recur. Some lessons we quickly learn from and move on while others present us the opportunity to assist or teach others. Sometimes I consider it a flaw of mine to be always reaching out to others, often neglecting myself. Conversely, deep within me is a voice of reason where I can put emotion aside and discover common sense.

Forgiveness appears to be a lesson that I have had to repeat over and over. I recall a friend of mine once reminding me that we can only control how we respond to a situation because in the end, we all answer to God.

I understand that men think and respond differently than women. I think I did what most women respond with—emotion providing for the needs of the children. I don't believe Steve knew how to be any different. I don't know his past, but sensed his insecurities behind that toughened exterior, and similar to Patti, his façade prevented others from coming too close. He needed to be in control at whatever cost. Perhaps he didn't know how to love or perhaps he considered his parents' divorce some sort of abandonment and his behavior was affected perversely.

Although the vow of marriage is "till death do us part," I don't believe that many of us make that commitment while expecting death to come prematurely. What I do know though is that somewhere inside of Steve, I am sure he misses my sister, I guess I don't know. I miss her physical presence almost every day of my life.

His experience of losing my sister, his wife, paralleled my grandfather's. Grandpa turned to alcohol, Steve turned inward. Unfortunately, we all had our own dysfunction, struggled to survive, and we had no energy left to love one another the way God intended.

I am thankful today to be alive to talk about my experiences and to have the ability to look inward and backward. The fortune of time has helped me to realize that I wasn't always able to see the bigger picture. I am now able to recognize the role I played in my environment. My protective bubble may have kept me safe, but it also kept me disconnected and oblivious to my surroundings. I can now see that I failed to see through the eyes of others. I am still evolving.

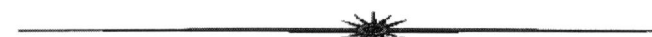

No one feels another's grief, so no one understands another's joy. People imagine they can reach one another. In reality they only pass each other by.

Frank Schubert

<u>Beating In Vain:</u>

    There are times when the heart, despite how much it works to compensate for faults in the system, just cannot succeed. In the case of a rupture in a large vessel for example, the type that occurs in a massive stroke, massive heart attack, or ruptured aneurysm the heart's efforts will be in vain.

    The heart's natural response to correct the situation is to increase its rate in a valiant effort to make up for the lost volume in the system. As blood continues to escape from the rupture, it pours out of the vessel, shifts into the tissues, and allows the blood pressure to plummet. Without blood in the system, the vital organs of the body including the brain, cannot be nourished. The heart will literally sacrifice itself in an effort to salvage the body. When the bleeding cannot be brought under control, the brain will shut down to preserve itself while the heart continues to fight, beating itself into its own final destiny.

    No one can predict the perfect life, the perfect path, or the perfect outcome. Life may simply be the luck of the draw or in a more positive outlook, merely a sequence of events that we are to learn and grow from. I used to refer to my life as a "series of unfortunate events," because I would feel like I was repeatedly beat on and knocked back down. I have since realized how very fortunate I really am. It seems that no matter how badly I may "bleed" from the beatings, somehow I have managed to overcome them, suffering only a few bruises along the way. Never has my bleeding

POTHOLES

gone entirely out of control and I've always somehow healed.

Dr. Stevenson came in bright and early in the morning and walked directly to the window. "You know, most people don't realize how much extra light there is if you open these up all the way. The windows go from floor to ceiling. I'd like to see them open every day. Let the sunshine in, it will help keep your spirits up," he told me.

I complied initially leaving the shades open for convenience; I couldn't reach them with my line in. It seemed to please Dr. Stevenson to come in each morning and talk about the view, but ultimately it was therapeutic for me. I welcomed the daylight sun as well as the city lights at night. If I woke in the middle of the night I could see the stars or sometimes fog. It was now peaceful there.

The beauty I could sometimes see from my hospital window would sometimes help me to forget about the tubes connected to my body and the monitors. I liked to sleep on my stomach but the tubing made it difficult. I learned to prop pillows around myself so that I could sleep more comfortably.

One night, I woke with my hand under my chin and my pillow was wet. *Ewe, gross,* I thought, believing I had drooled on it. I proceeded to turn my pillow over but in the moon's light spotted a dark spot on its edge. Realizing immediately it was blood, I used the call light for help. The overhead light was like a spotlight and I could barely see the person who entered my room. Squinting I tried to adjust. *I think I'm...* I didn't finish my thought as I saw her face grimace and she quickly exited the room. Until then I simply thought that maybe my P.A. line had loosened up, but seeing her reaction, knew differently. Within moments, there were four nurses lined up at the bedside. It reminded me of one of those movies where an aggressive individual is restrained.

"Your line is bleeding and we need to hold pressure on the site to stop it." A few failed attempts resulted in a call to another nurse from the Cardiac Intensive Care Unit.

Gary began to clean up some of the blood to allow him to visualize what was happening. "The sutures have come out and the line is loose, call the attending."

It took a little while to bring the bleeding under control.

"Thank goodness it's only a vein," I heard him say.

My immediate thought was, *Yeah my jugular vein!* Once he left, the nurses began to clean me up; the nurses, not the aides and it took a few moments to understand why.

Normally, the sight of blood doesn't usually bother me, but in this case it wasn't just a puddle, it was a pond and it was mine!

Blood extended around my pillow seeping across my shoulders and drained down the bed to my waistline. It was congealed around my neck and down the front of my gown. *No wonder,* I thought, *that aide left so quickly, I must've been quite a site to see in the middle of the night!*

After all this excitement I was alert, but still very tired. I wondered what woke me up in the first place but was so thankful I did. I feared what could've been.

Admittedly, I was unnerved and my patience shattered. I vowed that I was going to go back to sleep and not get out of bed for a week. This event caused my comfort level and confidence to be stripped. So many things had happened in the short time I was in the hospital. Things were just so unpredictable and all I really wanted to do then was curl up in a ball and cry. I had no one to comfort me, no one to hold me; my heart was bleeding in a much different sense. I now had mixed emotions about my safety and felt myself slipping back into being a lonely child. I remembered a technique that Kristyn taught me to feel comforted: I visualized myself as a child being lovingly held by myself as an adult. I was the one person I could always count on.

The child I saw was me at around the age of eight years of age, a time when my mom was alive and I felt safe. I called us "little Linda and big Linda." We would hug one another, rocking back and forth telling ourselves it would be O.K.

The next day Kristyn popped in to see me. She asked how my night was and how I felt about what I had just been through with the bleeding line.

"I am physically feeling my heart throw irregular beats and it concerns me. I am emotionally drained," I told her. "I sometimes feel the nurses aren't looking in on me often enough and something ominous may happen," I continued.

Kristyn let me know, "It's O.K. to feel the way you do Linda, and you are allowed to express your concerns." "You have endured so much," she comforted me.

I explained that though I often appear to be in control, sometimes that performance can be misleading to others.

She asked what part of me, what emotion was I feeling? Very quickly I was able to define it: "I am feeling unsafe, unprotected," I replied.

Immediately, she asked for a piece of paper and writing utensil. On the paper she wrote: "May I be happy and peaceful, may I feel healthy and strong, may I feel safe and protected, may I live with ease of mind and heart." "It is a mantra that I think may help... Repeat it as often as you need," she said as she handed me the paper.

It was an "Aha" moment! This theme affected me throughout my life and chronically repeated itself: safety and protection. Her words allowed me to explore my feelings from very deep within. She did not judge me; I didn't have to prove myself with her or pretend to be brave. I liked having her on my team. She was genuine, full of insight, and positive in thought and expression. She was like having your favorite fuzzy slippers: very welcomed on a difficult day!

I was able to calm, able to regroup, and was ready to move on. I was even able to laugh when my friends and family joked about my blood being the result of "the vampires in New England." Ironically I was still reading the *Twilight* series at the time and the comments were very appropriate!

Although the line was salvaged the night before, it wedged again, this made me increasingly nervous when the doctors came in with their purple gloves on. Imagine how relieved I was that they were able to correct it without removing it this time!

Dr. Stevenson told me, "The lines support cardiac monitoring and medication administration, but are an infection risk if kept in much more than seven to ten days."

I now understood why they changed them when they did yet noticed the longer I was there, the less diligent they were about removing them. My schedule however aligned nicely with my visits with Chris who now came every other weekend. I loved seeing the doctor's order that read, "P.A. line out Friday, husband visiting."

In preparation for Chris and Vince, I redressed Bessie and re-stuffed her telling her, "We both wanted to look our best."

The ABC news team came in for an interview and of course was quite interested in Bessie too. My new camera person was Valery. We spoke extensively about my story, spilling all my family secrets and what had brought me to this point in my life. It was exhausting, but I enjoyed her presence. She was genuinely interested and listened intently. Everything about her, including her body posture, indicated sincerity.

I felt well enough to walk a little in the halls with Chris and his dad when they arrived and even went to the cafeteria with them. Ironically the smell of the greasy food was nauseating so I declined needing anything, especially recalling Kenny's warning.

"Don't eat anything there. The food is fatty and salty and you will get sick!" He was adamant.

I simply didn't have the energy to feel sicker so I just ate my "hospital food" when we returned to my room. What a strange milestone it was to not want French fries which is my favorite food!

I truly enjoyed my visits and actually was so grateful that I learned to appreciate the sound of Chris' snoring. In fact I missed it! I envisioned each breath was like a wave going in and out of shore. It became a calm serenity and comforted me. I fell asleep to the sound instead of wanting to put a pillow over his head.

I was awakened from sound sleep a while later by Chris tapping me on my arm.

"Linda, do you have a tissue?" he asked.

I looked at him confused as I reached across my bed to get them. I expected him to blow his nose, but instead he twisted the tissues up and scrunched them in his ears. Apparently he didn't appreciate his dad's snoring! I was amused and fell back to sleep holding on to Chris and taking him in as much as I possibly could.

I learned to admire his dad for taking the seven-hour drives routinely so Chris could visit so soon after his surgery. I learned to appreciate the simple presence of the ones I love. I cherished those moments because they ended so quickly. Each time Chris and his dad left for home again it was painful, almost like another round in a prize fight; with each round you got more beaten, more tired, less eager to get back up. Despite this, I did get up, just like I had as a child.

I looked into his eyes seeing the same pain I was feeling as he prepared to leave. "I am going to cry," I informed him.

He gently squeezed by arms and nodded, "I know."

For the first time in my life no one was telling me not to! I had permission. I felt a weight had been lifted from my shoulders and I sobbed in his arms. I'm not sure if the grip he had on me was to console me or prevent me from seeing his tears, but I was engulfed in my own emotional thunderstorm.

After he left, I confined myself to my room trying to understand my pain, questioning God's intentions. I screamed inside my head, *I don't know what normal is!* I tried to comfort myself, struggled to breath, and finally told myself to stop it! Usually I have a rule about wallowing in self-pity: wallow for a few moments and then move on, but none of my normal coping tricks were effective. I knew it was because I had not allowed myself to love this way, to trust this way, nor to feel pain this way. It was uncharted territory. I needed time to explore it, digest it, and then allow myself to respond to what I felt.

I had so much intensity inside I wanted to jump around, jog, dance, hop, or whatever I could to release it, but didn't have the physical energy. I grabbed by iPod, shut the door, and began to sing my heart out.

Katherine was always right there to pick up my pieces when I fell apart. For the first time, I heard a phrase about "God's timing."

"God gives us what we need, not what we want," she said. It was the second time someone had said this to me. I wondered, "What does God want for me?" I spent a few hours in quiet contemplation after she left.

Shortly after, one of the nurses popped in and told me I might want to go down to Kenny's room. I was intrigued so I took a walk. When I reached his room, Kenny announced that he was going to get his heart. My sadness was gone suddenly to see that God was busy working on something very important at that moment. His family filled his room, everyone was ecstatic that the time had finally come. The energy was abounding. I was thrilled for Kenny as I stood in his room chatting with his family. I realized I was thrilled for each of them as well. They were a wonderfully dedicated and loving family.

I left his room and went to sit by the elevators to cry. I laid on the bench at the end of the corridor with the sun streaming in the window, and tears rolling down my cheeks. I was alone and I wished it were me going for surgery. Wrapped in so much emotion, I felt guilty.

Suddenly I felt a hand on my shoulder and heard my name. It was Dr. Ken. He sat down on the bench next to me and talked with me for a while. His hand was like a message from heaven at the perfect time. No, I was not alone, I had my friends and I had God.

A few days later, Geoff visited introducing me to Sheila, and his daughter. We sat in his room laughing at life and learning from one another's experiences. It was hard for me to imagine planning an event like a wedding when life looked so uncertain, but it was inspiring to hear. Geoff's heart came just a few days after Kenny's. Three of us had been blessed, and the rest of us remained.

On an enormously wonderful day, I was pleasantly surprised by a visit from my daughter Amanda, Keith her fiancé, my grandkids, my son Adam, and his girlfriend Jade. They came up to visit before Easter and I was thrilled to see them all. The nurses were very accommodating despite so many people visiting. We were packed into my room and had a great time. I took a lot of pictures on my cell phone of everyone sleeping in my bed but me, all tired from the long drive.

Amanda showed her creative streak and highlighted my hair. I had just enough I.V. tubing to reach the hand washing sink while the nurses tried to turn their heads the other way. It felt good to be pampered and did my heart a world of good. I was elated! They ordered pizza for me which I hadn't had in months! I cautiously ate the treacherous pizza, all the while, hearing Kenny's warning in my head, but thoroughly enjoyed it anyway. What a turn of events having my kids take care of me. I was grateful.

Ashtynne, my 2-year-old granddaughter, spent quite a bit of time in my lap coloring and playing with items I had in a "happy box" my friend Tena had sent. It was loaded with activities and came in quite handy. Engulfed in the simplicity of a child's innocence, the simple pleasure of coloring meant the world to me. At her young age, she seemed to sense my illness and remained cautious not to hurt me or pull any tubes. There was a deeply concerned look in her young blue eyes. I can't imagine what her little mind must have been thinking, but I assured her things would be alright. She was my little advocate, asking the nurses about the procedures they were doing for me.

Tanner who was only six-months-old had grown so much in the few months since I had seen him last. You forget how precious time is until you have lost it. He now had a few teeth and a brilliant smile. When I was holding him, he had gotten hold of the tubing on my neck with a death grip, the kind like when a baby grabs your hair. As I clutched his hand, Amanda and Jade sprung to my rescue. I know we all panicked but all turned out fine. It gave us a great laugh afterward.

It was a wonderfully uplifting visit, yet seeing them leave was a critical turning point in my determination to get this process over with. I was now angry that I was missing out on my life, missing seeing my boys at home, missing my family, wanting to see my grandbabies grow!

Easter was a difficult day. It was my first holiday alone, unless St. Patrick's Day counts. I had been elevated to a wonderful feeling of bliss with my family and now I was alone again. It's a long way to fall. I cried uncontrollably most of the day, feeling incredibly helpless. Somewhere I read that, "Tears are the relief valve for the heart," and I recanted that I was relieving a lot of pressure that day! That day, I hit an all time low. I closed my hospital room door in anger for the first time since I'd been in the hospital. I agonized seeing all the families together and hearing the children in the halls.

Once again, heaven intervened. There was a knock on my door. It was Kenny's family: Nancy, Daniel, and Nicole, stopping by to let me know how he was doing after his surgery. I was amazed at their kindness and thought about what a selfless act it was on their part to stop by to see me. I cried when they left, but in gratitude for their visit. Soon after, there was another knock at the door. This time it was Dr. Ken's wife, Surrinder. She stopped at the store and brought me a chocolate bunny for Easter. It didn't have the crazy eyes like Wilson though, but I was consumed with gratitude for her kindness. We had a nice chat and I was so grateful she took the time to pop by.

Again, I wept after she left, this time from a different emotional level.

As I tried to compose myself, I asked the nurses if a special dinner was provided for the holiday. The answer was, "No." I was disappointed. This was "the year without Easter" in my eyes. There were none of the holiday traditions to look forward to.

I fell asleep that day out of pure emotional exhaustion. I woke, to a plate of food on my bedside table. Someone had brought me Easter dinner from home! I later learned it was Lauren's family. I began to cry again, happy tears, almost uncontrollably. It is hard to describe how far I had come in this journey. I had gone from a frightened, orphaned child to someone who had three separate families who cared for me. I was sort of adopted, and God gave me what I needed that day. Looking at this gift of love on my table, I was overwhelmed with joy!

When the doctors popped in, they asked if my family had been in. I began to cry as I explained that my family was back in Buffalo. The doctor looked at me puzzled. "Why are you crying?" she asked.

As a nurse I know not to ask "why" questions because it creates a defensive response. I grew instantly angry because I was already upset and felt I shouldn't need to justify my feelings to her. It should've been self-explanatory. Instead she assumed I was depressed and asked me if I needed medication. I looked at her in disbelief! I wanted to scream, *are you kidding me?*

They charted that my mood needed to be monitored! *Unbelievable!* I thought.

The next morning I had recharged and was feeling good. I rearranged my room a little and counted my blessings. My heart was no longer heavy nor yearning for what it couldn't have. Things were in check…at least for the day.

Reflection:

I once read a poem and I'm not sure where but it was about a little boy talking to God. In it the boy inquires about the value of a million dollars and God replies, "It is like a penny to me." The boy asks about a million years and God replies, "It's like a second to me." At the end the boy asks God for a million dollars and God replies, "In a second."I remember reading this as a patient and realizing how profound it was. I realized it was typical for me to want everything right here and now, but for the first time I realized God had a different timetable and I would need to be patient. I truly recognized the abundance of blessings that I had and was diligently counting them. It was also at this time I recognized that getting a heart was not a given and it would be God's will. I prayed now for the best possible outcome knowing it was out of my hands. Letting go and letting God is not an easy task, but one that is necessary to grow.

Weeping may endure for the night, but joy comes in the morning.

-Psalm 30:5 NKJV

Chapter 8
The Deceptive Heart

The heart is about the size of our fist and grows at the same rate as our bodies. It is a hollow muscular organ that pumps blood, the fluid of life, through an extensive network of blood vessels that if stretched end-to-end would extend over 60,000 miles. Amazingly, for each pound of fat that we are overweight the circulatory system creates another collateral mile of vessels to nourish it.

As a child grows, his or her personality traits develop also at a predictable rate. If a child's needs are met, that child will develop a network of coping skills that supports that child's well-being and extends throughout that child's lifetime. For a child, feeling loved is his or her lifeline to which there is no replacement. Without love, a child may seek inappropriate or unhealthy relationships or may even find an escape through substance abuse.

I have always held a special place in my life for my sister Joyce I guess because I felt we were all one another had. We were born less than 13 months apart, which made us like twins. I felt responsible for the two of us since I was older. I was scrawny and gaunt; she had a glow about her. Her cheeks were rosy and full and in general Joyce resembled a cherub. She was taller than I; more jovial by all accounts and always appeared to seem content. I, on the other hand, was more serious than my almost twin and certain discontent ran through my veins. The contrast could be seen in our eyes. We each had brown eyes; hers were almond with a golden ring around her iris and playful black flecks near her pupil, mine were a dark, determined, serious brown with black flecks. Our smiles were similar except her teeth were squarer like "Chicklets" and she had a cute curve to the corner of her lips. I envied the clarity of her skin and the beauty mark near her nose. I always thought she was the pretty one.

Joyce had a soft plumpness about her for as long as I can remember and it remained part of her character throughout our lives. She sucked her thumb to nurture herself, I guess to comfort her, since our mother was not the type of mother to hold us. To pacify her as a child, the adults who cared for her fed her, so she learned to eat in order to cope. Food provided comfort for her and was probably easier for my mother to provide than maternal warmth. I felt like I was the only one who loved her. My earliest memories involved protecting Joyce, especially when my mom and Wally left us alone, as they often did. Those nights without a babysitter were frightening.

"Don't worry Joycie; we can go into our fort to sleep." I would console her and we would head into our safe place under the china cabinet. Sometimes, I would bring a knife and place it under my pillow. Maybe fear caused my imagination to run away from me, but I was there to protect my sister against whatever the night could bring. I was relieved that I never had to use it. The sadness I carried as an adult is in the knowledge that the instability of my childhood days was reinforced by my mother. She inconsistently provided for us then. Outwardly, I was surviving the lack of attention. Joyce, however, became an empty shell who filled her void with food.

One night we were left alone and we were hungry. We weren't old enough to read or to know how to prepare food, so we dialed phone numbers from the pictures in the phone book. I told Joyce not to worry.

"I will press some numbers, just like Mommy does, and when the doorbell rings, pizza will arrive," I told her.

We waited in our fort. Well, I was right, the doorbell rang, but the pizza did not come, only the Police. Wally and Mom were directly behind them. I can't say it was the last time we were left alone, but it was the last time we dialed strange numbers from the phone book.

Into adulthood, using food for comfort, further led Joyce to struggles with many self-esteem issues. She draped herself in the joy of material things, expensive clothes and fine jewelry, pampering herself to replace her unmet needs with "things." As time passed, Joyce began to pattern herself after my step-sister Roberta, which was uncharacteristic for my little sister. I often wondered if she held the same secret that I did; the dark secrets of having Wally abuse her as he did me. As she grew into an adult, it was a question I would never ask her, even when the time came when she was ready to marry.

After years of struggles and disappointment, Joyce met Daniel and fell in love. They were married on the Fourth of July, 1987. It was a beautiful wedding that the entire family participated in: Independence Day seemed fitting. My sister Patti sang and played the piano as Joyce walked down the aisle. Joyce wore an incredibly beautiful gown drenched with sparkling sequins that complimented the glow on her face. She was absolutely stunning. I admired Daniel's love for her despite her weight issues. "Her little feet have such an important job to carry her around," he would endearingly tell us.

As a couple they were very laid back, but not organized or disciplined. Daniel rarely kept a job long enough to support them, often he was injured with one medical problem or another, but somehow they got by. He was like a cat with nine lives and had exhausted most of them. It always seemed that there was something underlying that was not quite right, but it was a situation that I just could not put my finger on. The problem echoed Patti and Steve's marriage. I told myself that my sisters' marriages were dysfunctional. I told myself that my marriage was so much better than theirs, but it really wasn't. Regardless of stumbling blocks, we were there for one another.

One night, Joyce and Daniel's home burnt down. Despite the trauma of losing all their possessions, I was so relieved to learn they were alright. I couldn't fathom losing her. Without a place to stay, Ray and I opened our home to them.

In our cramped quarters, we all got to know one another quite extensively. They lived with us until they found a new home. In that time it became apparent to me that married life changes who you are; or at least it had changed my sisters for sure and probably me as well.

Joyce and Daniel ended up renting the house he grew up in. In all their married years they never owned a home. It was a cute white ranch with red brick accents and black shutters. It had three bedrooms and a spacious yard adorned with flower beds and a babbling brook. I would go there with my kids and work furiously in their yard; possibly attempting to organize the clutter as if that could stop the confusion in our lives. Joyce and her husband acquired several rental properties during their marriage, despite not having stable incomes. They were all in poor condition, just plain dirty, but provided income none the less. It was income that only Daniel had control over.

As time passed, Joyce and Daniel were blessed with two children, Lauren and Perry. I was so proud to hold her as Lauren's Godmother when she was baptized. She became stunningly beautiful as she grew with long, dark, silky hair and beautiful olive-colored skin, and almond shaped eyes. Her beauty radiated from deep within. Lauren's mannerisms were shy and gentle through every childhood growing pain, it was rare to hear her complain; about anything.

Perry, seeming to be a little more of a challenge, was demanding and sometimes aggressive. To his parents' surprise, he was born eight years after Lauren. As a baby, Perry was angelic, with nice round features, dark brown eyes and thick curly eye lashes. Holding him was challenging as he usually seemed restless and discontent. We knew that Perry was different, but it was just one more time we did not say anything to each other. We just relished in the fact that we were all adults who raised and loved our children together.

POTHOLES

We weren't going to let anything interfere as we made the best of our days then. That time will always remain cherished for all of us.

It would be years before a formal diagnosis of Autism would be made, yet it made no difference. Perry was always special and we loved him for who he was. Often, we all got together and played or went somewhere fun. I thought it would always be that way. We all did what sisters do, babysit each other's kids, went to the beach, and picnicked in the park.

Joyce was my daughter Erin's godmother and it was a beautiful world. We were the godparents for each other's children. We were the sisters that stood side by side, sometimes complaining about husbands, sharing dinners together when they did not come home and holding each other up, in good times as well as in bad. Actually, it seemed that the sisterhood was more powerful than our marriages, but even the sisterhood had its own "potholes."

As a teenager, my daughter Erin gravitated towards Joyce instead of me and I knew why. There were no boundaries with Joyce. Erin learned to manipulate Joyce when she couldn't get her way with me. Our roles were getting confused. Erin pitted Joyce and me against each other, as if we were two parents in the midst of a bad divorce. I fought to keep Erin with me while Joyce was taking Erin to have a belly piercing and tattoos, against my wishes.

I fought for Erin, as I had for Joyce when we were young. Rage simmered within me as the insults and statements of how I was too strict continued. It was so difficult to be effective as a parent when Joyce undermined my authority. Still, I could not leave her. I could not move away from Joyce, my beautiful cherub sister who draped herself with jewels. Perhaps, she provided stability for me too.

So, there we were, all our families, almost merged as one. We would raise our children together in this less than perfect world. My sisters were my best friends. At the time, and I couldn't understand how other families could allow trivial events to ever separate them. I had it great I believed.

I have heard it said that money is the root of all evil. The bitter truth became the flesh eating savage leading Joyce and I into the next chapter of our lives. After Daniel won over two million dollars in a lawsuit from a construction injury, I was thrilled beyond imagination for them but not knowing the dangers that lurked in excessive amounts of money. Undetected evil crept into our lives. What should have been a good thing became horrific!

Together, Joyce and Daniel purchased a bar and restaurant called Ragoo's. We spent days upon days cleaning, organizing, and painting in preparation for their place to open. I was so proud of what my sister had accomplished. It was a dream that had come true for her, and for the first time in her life, I believed she would be all right. The bar itself was very cozy with a beautiful oak bar and tables, tastefully colored stained glass lamps, and a calming color scheme of beige, burgundy, and forest green . It also had quaint brick accent arches that separated the bar from the dining area. Joyce had been developing incredible culinary skills and ran a great kitchen.

Soon after purchasing Ragoo's, they gave up their rented home to live in the tiny two bedrooms, 400 square foot apartment above the bar. Daniel said, "It will save us money." Joyce remained the dutiful wife and moved despite objection from their children. Perry complained crying, "I don't want my back yard to be a parking lot!" I thought that was pretty insightful for a six-year-old to identify this as a problem. To me, it was a mistake raising your family there: too close to the bar scene, too convenient for alcoholism, and a breeding ground for dysfunction, abuse, and violence.

Yet Joyce followed Daniels's lead; just as a defective gene would cause a heart to become diseased without warning, so too would the restaurant cause another kind of disease within my family.

Joyce at first seemed to thrive while running the bar. She took command and was very successful. When I'd visit, a smile stretched across her face as she'd boast about the fact that she was even losing weight. "I've lost fifty pounds since we opened," she would rejoice in her hurried way. "I am very proud of you," I would tell her. Joy abounded in her presence and she seemed to want to share her good fortune. She purchased beautiful jewelry of platinum bands and diamonds each costing over ten thousand dollars. I must admit that I was in awe, having never owned a piece of jewelry costing over more than a few hundred dollars.

One evening, Joyce walked to the table I was sitting at with my friends and took off one of her rings. "Here, I want you to have this."

"Why?" I inquired, "That is your ring."

"Because you are my sister and I want you to have nice things too," she replied. Handing the ring back, I declined of course, though secretly flattered by the gesture.

"I can't allow myself to accept such a generous offer. Your life has been difficult and you deserve everything that you get. I love you sister." After saying that to her she smiled, slid the ring on her finger and gave me a hug before walking away.

The bar was a place where we had adult fun. I tried to support my sister by patronizing her business during sporting events along with some of my friends. We focused on the positive, delighted in Joyce and Daniel's great fortune until one evening my friend Carmen joined me at the bar. She noticed things were not what they seemed and Carmen hinted that something was wrong.

It was at Ragoo's where my sister threw a surprise 40th birthday party for me. She lured me there by asking me to bartend for a few hours. I had no previous intention of spending my birthday there, but Joyce seemingly was in a bind and of course I set out to help her. That's what sisters do! Having a surprise birthday party thrown just for me was one of the most incredibly genuine and selfless gestures anyone had ever done for me, and I was ecstatic. I was thrilled to have my sister, thankful for our relationship and on top of the world. It seemed we were both at great points in our lives.

Daniel, on the other hand, pickled himself in alcohol that night, was a very angry drunk, and in fact as usual, was abusive to my sister and the kids. When he was drunk, he knew no boundaries. My birthday was no exception. A day that had started with all the love and excitement you would see on television shows like Happy Days or The Cosby's, shows in which families celebrated one another. The beginning of the party remains one of my fondest memories. The end of my party though more resembled Stephen King's, The Shining, where the lead character becomes psychotic.

    I couldn't understand why my sister stayed in that situation. Police involvement was often necessary. Then, rumblings about cocaine abuse and drug trafficking began to circulate. I didn't believe any of it, until my daughter Erin confided that she walked in on Daniel in the kitchen at the bar doing lines of cocaine off the counter top. She was bartending that evening and as the night progressed he became increasingly violent. At three-thirty in the morning, I woke to Erin's phone call pleading for help. She asked me to come to the bar and remove Joyce and Daniel's children from the apartment above the bar. Imagine that. At her young eighteen years of age, she was being the responsible one. I don't recall where my sister was that evening, but it mimicked my childhood memories of being alone; fearful of what may happen, yet void of her. The world in which we were all together seemed to come apart so quickly. My heart was now fragile and it wouldn't be long before it would shatter.

    The next day when I spoke with Joyce about the whole thing, she only admitted to Daniel being a casual drug user and claimed she wasn't threatened by it. I didn't understand the concept of "casual" and in my eyes it was illegal, habit-forming, and almost always led to a devastating outcome. I wondered why she wasn't protecting her children as a mother is supposed to. She herself denied any wrong doing other than an occasional drink. It was mind boggling how callus, unscathed, and accepting she seemed to appear.

Daniel's violent behavior often overlapped into the business. There were days the bar and restaurant would be thriving and Daniel would snap. He would decide to start smashing bottles of alcohol throughout the room often scaring customers away. I later learned that the "after hours" parties rocked with illegal activity when the bar closed and the word around town was Ragoo's was a fun place before 2 a.m. I didn't understand why my sister put her family in jeopardy with such chaos. I really did not realize that Joyce was into the chaos herself. I was so naive and trusting of her.

The next time Erin called me to the bar in the middle of the night to rescue the kids, I had had enough. When I arrived, I threatened to call the police. My threats were met by a confrontation by everyone in the bar who pleaded with me not to. I wondered what was wrong with all of these people. It was so confusing to me. I guess I just couldn't process the fact that everyone seemed misguided but me. I wondered why I was the only *car driving with four wheels while they all had three, but I seemed like the odd ball!*

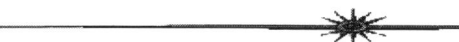

The violence continued and I again was awakened by a late night phone call fearing the worst. Joyce was frantic. "Linda you have to come right away. Daniel fell down the stairs and he's not moving."

"Is he breathing?" I asked.

"Yes, but I'm afraid he may be paralyzed." We had a fight and he was hurting me in front of the kids. He lost his balance and fell," she reported.

"Call an ambulance and I'll come get the kids," I told her.

"No, I'll just see if he gets up. I'll call you back," she said.

Admittedly, despite how incomprehensible each event was, each more unbelievable than the other, Daniel never went to the hospital. I later learned that they indeed had a fight, but it was Lauren who shoved him down the stairs protecting her mother. She was fourteen.

Finally, Joyce agreed to move out of the apartment above the bar to preserve a more normal lifestyle and obtained a restraining order against Daniel. I was relieved that she seemed to have her priorities in order. She would later tell stories of Daniel accusing her of embezzling his money, being investigated by the banks and having her assets frozen. He seemed to have a sick hold on her and she had a "fatal attraction" toward him. I couldn't defend her; I could no longer believe her.

A few months after my birthday, Joyce asked me to watch Perry while she attended a social event with the local bar owners. Lauren stayed with some friends. That whole night Daniel rang my phone looking for her. He was seemingly drunk and slurring his words. I knew to remain calm with him when he was like this because he would continue to call and each call would get increasingly belligerent, and it did. I knew his violent history; I was afraid of him, afraid for the kids, and afraid for my sister. Despite the restraining order, Daniel still seemed to know many details of my sister's life and whereabouts.

Joyce did not come home that night and Daniel's calls continued into the next day. I became infuriated that her irresponsibility was now invading my home. Daniel showed up at my house asking where Joyce was and I had no answers for him. I had no idea where she was and I began to grow concerned about her safety.

Enraged at my lack of information, Daniel began an almost ritualistic purging of all kinds of wrong doings on my sister's part. "Did you know your sister is a drug addict? Did you know she's probably using you to watch the kids while she's out getting high? How does that make you feel? I don't know what to do anymore. She's been to rehab and hid it from you. She's a liar!" Daniel went on and I asked him to stop.

"I can't listen to this anymore. It is my sister," I told him. My head was spinning.

"You think you know her, you don't! She's a thief. Did you know she stole $30,000 from our bank account? Do you know that she's so strung out she doesn't send the kids to school? Is that your sister too?"

I couldn't think straight and was grateful his cell phone rang interrupting his tangent. I didn't want any of it to be true. I just wanted someone to wake me from the nightmare. There were so many lies; so many lies.

I thought, *I'm going to be ill*.

When he got off the phone he looked at me with a determined grin.

"It was your sister. She wants to meet me at the house," he told me.

"Daniel, don't go, there's the restraining order," I pleaded, fearing what may happen.

Before I finished the words the front door had slammed and he was gone. My stomach sank and I couldn't think quick enough to react. I wanted to follow him to ensure my sister was safe, but I had to stay with Perry.

Meanwhile, Lauren had returned home to Joyce's apartment. She called looking for her mother. I knew she was safe for the moment.

"Lauren, just stay put, Mom should be home shortly," I told her as calmly as I could. When my phone rang again, it was Daniel. He told me I needed to come to their old house right away because I needed to see what my sister was up to.

"She's smoking crack and you need to come so I can prove it to you once and for all," he insisted. Feeling defeated and wanting an end to the drama, I asked my daughter Amanda who had recently come home, to watch Perry. I left never thinking what might happen. For me, I just wanted Daniel's psychotic episodes to stop. I believed I was rushing to help her. Maybe I was just plain desperate for the truth; for any of it to finally make sense.

When I arrived, Daniel gestured for me to come in and placed his hand over his lips indicating I should be quiet. He motioned me toward the bathroom door which was locked and he jimmied the door open with a butter knife. He was prepared. In the first glimpse I saw the back of my sister's head bent over the toilet as if she were ill. She dragged herself to her feet and stumbled out of the bathroom looking incredibly disheveled. As she staggered toward us, I saw my sister in a way I would have never imagined. Her bleached blonde hair tussled like she had been electrocuted. Her makeup was smeared, pupils were dilated, and her clothing hung off her shoulders as if she'd been in a fight. Her nose was running with a little blood from her left nostril that met her lips. She was strung out. I was terrified and repulsed.

Daniel yelled about her being high on crack and proceeded to show me a spoon. "This is what she cut it with," he said. He proceeded to show me a plastic cola bottle duct-taped with a straw. "Here's the pipe she used to smoke it!" He was determined to get his point across.

I was speechless! She looked at him, her eyes narrowed into slits. "I hate you," she hissed.

She didn't acknowledge me, and didn't wipe the drainage from under her nose. He continued to yell at her and his voice seemed to fade in my mind as I forced myself to speak.

I asked her, "Joyce, what am I supposed to do with this?"

She positioned her hands and shrugged her shoulders as if to say, "I don't care." At that very moment, the world seemed to spin out of control and stop all at the same time. I realized I was in an incredibly bad situation where I had to do something immediately, but what? My heart was beating so hard I could feel the blood throb through my head. I couldn't call for help; there was a violated restraining order, people were under the influence of illegal substances, and paraphernalia was in the house. I couldn't call the police, I was afraid of how this could get manipulated against me. I was afraid of what they were capable of. I couldn't trust either of them and I had Perry at my house.

Daniel then handed me the phone and suddenly I was speaking to Child Protective Services (CPS) on the line. I spoke with them explaining the situation, unsure how the phone dialed. I didn't realize until later that Daniel handed me a dialed phone as if he planned the outcome. Was this some form of abuse or revenge? Was it a deliberate attempt to hurt her? I didn't know. At the time, my emotions ran high. This was my baby sister! I had never anticipated an experience this awful could ever have happened to any of us.

I was asked by CPS to keep the kids and file for temporary custody. I did this with a heavy heart (unaware that my sister and Daniel had an extensive history with CPS). No one would ever want to be the bearer of that type of pain and knowingly hurt their only lifeline as I was forced to do. I went to the apartment to get Lauren before heading back to my home for Perry. Joyce was there and Lauren was an emotional wreck when I arrived. I have no idea what occurred before I arrived and I could barely bring myself to look at Joyce.

Lauren then locked herself in her room screaming in shrill tones at her mother. "You don't care about us!" she shrieked.

She wanted nothing to do with me. I was numb as I pleaded with her to open the door and come with me. My sister showed no emotion and she remained in her kitchen. I felt helpless. Once I was able to get into Lauren's room, I found a hardened shell of hatred. I told her that we needed to go to my house for awhile.

There is no life lesson that could've prepared me for the loss and devastation this experience brought. The one person in my life that I thought I knew better than anyone else, my connection to life, and the constant I thought I could always count on had disintegrated.

In court the lies and disbelief continued. The pain became excruciating as my wounds ground with salt. I sat silently as the lawyers referred to me as the "estranged aunt" and referred to "attempts to extort money." I literally looked around the court room to see who they were talking about. It was like I was hit with a brick...they were talking about me! They were the finest lawyers each one of them had hired against one another: against me.

For the next six-months the kids stayed with my family. Everyone had been torn apart, and even my daughter Erin found that she couldn't cope with her world crumbling into this nightmare. Her Aunt Joyce who was her "Goddess," had turned out to be a "druggie." She packed up and moved to Florida to get as far away as she could.

It would be years later that I learned that my sister also supplied my children and hers with drugs: incomprehensible to this day.

Heartbreak was no stranger to me at this time. Ray and I were finally at a breaking point in our lives. The strain from each day seemed to push us further away from each other. For Joyce and Daniel, each toxicology test continued to be positive which delayed the kids from returning to their home. It was a no-win situation, and for Ray and I the only thing holding us together was fear of falling apart. Nothing was stable, nothing was sacred.

My sister and her husband were back together, played the "good parent role" with their choices, while Ray and I were the "bad parents." They got the kids on weekends for all the fun activities, long enough to unravel any forward progress we had attained. In that time they vacationed in Las Vegas and the Dominican Republic, places they could obtain drugs. Perry called us "the stupid family" and I made light of it singing it to the tune of the *Adams Family*.

Perry had multiple behavioral issues that needed to be dealt with including violence, anger, and impulsivity. One day he got mad and hit me with a rock. As blood drained from the split in my forehead, there was no remorse in his face.

"Look at what you've done!" I yelled at Perry.

"Mom!" I heard Adam call from behind me. "Go get help, I will handle Perry," he said.

The wound was able to be managed without stitches but my emotions were scarred.

Behavioral issues continued daily and Perry refused to sleep at night. His routines were engrained: up most of the night, sleep during the day. We were run ragged while Joyce and Daniel went on partying. I knew I needed a break or I would be heading for a nervous breakdown. Ray adamantly refused to accept any further custody under these circumstances. The kids were returned to their home under the guided support and supervision of their paternal grandmother who kept an eye on Joyce and Daniel.

At the next court date, Ray spoke up. "Your honor, having these kids has disrupted our lives. Perry has needed extensive therapy, tutoring, and supports in school. He had missed over 100 days and was so far behind we have had to obtain tutors. We are forced to allow visitation which is further damaging to any forward progress we have made. We know it is not the best thing for them, but we are powerless here." "We are no longer willing to continue to care for these kids. Their needs are too great, and we are receiving no assistance with their care. We can no longer manage." Ray had made the decision and it hurt!

What we both realized is that the system had failed us. My sister and her husband became part-tIme parents while we struggled day-to-day.

When the kids went back, Joyce and Daniel were mandated to therapy; Ray and I were beyond treatment. Our world was broken and it would take years to recover from both the broken trust, and time that could never be recaptured. I suppose the phase "up in smoke" is probably appropriate for the two million dollars that was now gone. Beyond that, the whole thing was painfully senseless and greater than my other losses. Joyce has never seemed to be able to close the door to her life with Daniel, even after they divorced years later. His dysfunction has a gripping, suffocating hold on her. Addiction robs the soul.

Reflection:

Initially when I looked back at everything that occurred, I blamed myself for not recognizing there were problems, for not identifying the signs of substance abuse and addiction. I could've never comprehended that drugs could overshadow the love a mother could have for a child or the bonds shared among siblings raised among such adversity...never could I have imagined.

I now am able to recognize that among all the dysfunction in our lives, Joyce was rarely nurtured lovingly or appropriately. Her needs were met with alternatives to comfort, initially food, and later alcohol and drugs. She chose the path of so many: escape instead of using her "collateral circulation;" reaching out for help. I guess it shouldn't have surprised me knowing she had the deck stacked against her just like I did. I pondered what made the difference in the paths we chose or if there is a life lesson here. Sometimes life lessons are painful. If there is one thing I hope to accomplish, it is that I am able to help someone else though his or her own experience because of the wisdom I have gained through my own.

I have since forgiven my sister yet remain cautiously optimistic about her journey. Despite the devastation, despite the pain, despite it all harboring anger was hurting me.

I felt guilty for having been so wrapped up in my world that I did not pay attention to my lifeline, my only surviving sister; the one person I loved more than most anyone else. I have since forgiven myself recognizing that I really played no role in my sister's adult choices. I have forgiven her knowing that living within an entangled web of painful memories would destroy me and that her healing was a path she would need to venture alone.

From it all, I am thankful that my sister discovered the strength to recover from her addiction, had the ability to regain sole custody of her children, and had the strength to recognize that in order to have a life; she needed to close the book on her past, including her marriage. For her it has been a rocky road.

With time all wounds can heal, but that doesn't prevent the scars from being a constant reminder of a battle from long ago. I pray her children will also heal and be able to forgive.

*Grief can't be shared. Everyone carries it alone.
His own burden, his own way.*

Anne Morrow Lindberg

Bypassing the Heart: Vein stripping

As the body ages the heart works against forces which oppose it. The kidneys may work less efficiently causing a back up of blood that can cause distention in the veins or fluid overload when returning to the heart. The heart can become congested causing it to work harder against more volume. If allowed to continue, the lungs and other body systems may be adversely affected. Fluid in the lungs can make it difficult to breathe and when left untreated, could cause one to drown or suffocate.

As the clock of life ticks on, the responsibilities of raising a family, working, and maintaining day-to-day activities seem insurmountable. We live in a fast-paced, demanding society in which life sometimes gets away from us. While nurturing others we often neglect ourselves.

If we are fortunate, we have the support of a loving spouse or family to support us or balance it all. As children become older, their needs grow greater, more complicated, and they begin to understand the difference between wanting and needing. As these lessons surface, we learn to make valuable choices for both those who depend on us and for ourselves. If we don't take care of ourselves, our ability take care of others can become impaired or we can become depleted.

As a parent lacking support, over time, I grew weary and impatient. There was neither outlet nor magic fix. I found that I had no option other than to persevere. I knew there would be a light at the end of the tunnel. Eventually, I became smothered by my own "fluid overload" and knew that I needed to make a change to preserve my own life.

By now I had mastered the layout of my hospital room and decorated as tastefully as I could, have been in the hospital for so many weeks. I often moved my bed to whatever placement allowed me the most freedom. This meant that I could use my bathroom when I wanted to as long as no one caught me! I was ecstatic and very self-reliant; something that was comfortable to me. I was back!

I had a refrigerator in my room to store the goodies in that people brought me and saved them to share. Sometimes Jill, one of the nurses, would stop to visit in the evening and we would enjoy a good conversation over tea. Often, I would simply enjoy the quiet. I learned which light switches kept the room softly lit creating a calm ambience. I was at peace with myself, at peace with God, ready for whatever was to come. Many people who came in would comment on the calm presence in my room. It seemed to have a soothing effect on everyone who came by. It helped me to feel some sense of control of my environment while I surrendered everything else. One morning and I could sense a little tension in the air about the fact that I was so actively independent in my room. I got a fearful sense that something was brewing. Danielle explained, "The doctors are concerned that you could get hurt and in your condition are just doing too much. They think you should return to the previous level of activity."

As a nurse, I understood dignity of risk. I explained, "I would be more than happy to sign a waiver or be evaluated for safety, if necessary, but feel no reason to change."

I was mentally alert and aware of complications that could occur. I felt this was fair, and I was doing well. This was what was portrayed to the next shifts. I was able to enjoy my freedom one more day.

The next morning the buzz continued and tension surmounted.

"Do me a favor," Dr. Lewis asked, "just take it easy and don't discuss with other people what you are capable of doing."

I agreed. A few minutes later a very determined charge nurse came in my room with Dr. Lewis. She had a white binder in her hands. She demanded his attention and was pointing to a page in the book as if I wasn't present. "It's in the policy manual; patients with a P.A. cannot have bathroom privileges!"

Though aware of what was occurring, and afraid my freedom was to be taken away I was more offended by her approach than the topic. I was so proud of myself for being resourceful enough to create this independence in my room, and now feared it would be lost. Even more so, I was insulted. I found the scenario very unprofessional.

After they left my room, I sat feeling like a scorned child, as if "I was waiting for the other shoe to drop." Moments later, my nurse Danielle came in looking as though she were going to cry. She apologized to me saying, "I'm sorry but I can no longer allow you to use the bathroom because we have a policy against it." I felt bad that she had been sent in to do the "dirty work" for the others. I started to cry. I know that sounds silly, but being there in that room brought so little pleasure that the simplest things brought joy. It hurt when that joy was ripped away.

Sometimes it seemed as though patterns from my childhood continued to repeat themselves. I felt constantly backed up against the wall and challenged on the most primitive, juvenile things just to prove myself. The struggles I endured as a child to maintain my place in my world would normally force me go into fight mode, but here in the hospital I couldn't. I had no choice and physically there wasn't enough fight left in me. I guess accepting defeat in my best interest was a new lesson in humility. We are always learning, always being tested. It is how we grow.

I immediately developed a dislike for the doctor and nurse who I felt threatened by and considered cowardly. Anger filled my inner being which was counterproductive.

Later the doctor came back into my room, both to tell me himself that I could not use the bathroom, and to apologize for the outdated policy that adversely affected people like me. By the power of his simple gesture, I had forgiveness in my heart. He was truly genuine. I told him, "I owe you an apology because I judged you unfairly."

He seemed quite surprised and thanked me for taking the step to keep an open doctor-patient relationship. All was forgiven and it was very cleansing.

Once again I began to turn my energy into determined creativity. Instead of using the bathroom, I made one. I put the commode in the corner and placed it where the curtain could surround it thus making an impromptu bathroom. I hung a picture above the commode and used the basket on the I.V. pole for toiletries such as hand antiseptic and personal products. I also took some tape and created a toilet paper holder on the wall. It didn't have running water, but I felt vindicated!

In the meantime, I learned that Dr. Ken had been called for a heart on not one but two occasions, but never had surgery. I needed to understand what had happened and walked to his room when I was freed from my line. I had learned so much about him, his wife Surrinder, and his entire family. They were very proud, yet very private, and when in each others' presence there was a remarkable resilience. I was awestruck by their dedication to one another and seemingly endless love.

On a few occasions, when I was fortunate enough to have been in the right place at the right time, I was able to be a surrogate family member, a confident. I cherished the purpose I found and was blessed by the opportunity to know that they were comfortable with me and I with them, sharing a few tear-filled moments. We all seemed to rotate our moments of weakness.

When I went into his room there was a quiet calm. They always seemed happy to see me. I asked if the rumor about getting called for a heart was true. Dr. Ken and his wife talked about their experiences. On the first occasion when Dr. Ken was called for a heart, he was a" back up" meaning if another primary candidate didn't work out, he would be the recipient. Once again I felt that double-edged sword.

To me it represented that he had made it to the top of his list and his turn would be fast approaching, yet I still waited. I then evaluated his intense disappointment attached to not getting that organ, the sheer let down. I sat in quiet contemplation.

There were so many moments that made me stop dead in my tracks and wonder what my path would be, could be. The anticipation was mounting. I worried about Dr. Ken. I watched his heart monitor, knowing there was little left for him. It frightened me and deep within I wished for his miracle of life before my own. I wanted their love to have a future. I prayed that God would listen.

The second time a heart became available he was the primary candidate. When everything was completely arranged, Dr. Ken was prepared for surgery. While in the operating room, a final inspection of the organ was performed revealing there was what is referred to as "vegetation" on the heart. I pictured green moss growing on it because of the term used. The organ was unusable. I couldn't imagine waiting all that time, being transported to the O.R., and then hearing that news…

When I spoke to him his voice was calm and very grateful. "I'm glad that this was discovered before they opened me up for surgery, and before the heart was transplanted. It wasn't the right time for me," he said calmly.

I had a great deal of respect for his attitude, his outlook, patience, and insight. The outcome was favorable at the time and more importantly, I was happy my "adopted family" was still safely intact.

Later that day, Kristyn stopped by. As always, I was thrilled to see her. "Hey, I need a favor. There is a female patient on the floor in a similar situation as you. Would you be open to talking to her?" Kristyn asked.

"Of course," I told her.

"Her name is Julie, in case she stops in." Kristyn continued, "One more thing, I'd like your opinion, I am preparing for a presentation for a class I am taking and wanted to touch base with you on your perspective of the transplant experience thus far," she said.

I was happy to receive the gift of purpose from her once again. "Let me think about it. Can I give you feedback tomorrow?" She nodded and left after a brief visit. I thought about it overnight and gave her what I thought was a cleverly woven representation spun with a very typical version of current times.

When she returned the next day I was prepared.

"Life as a transplant patient is very much like the current world of electronics: fast-paced, ever-changing, and too busy to acknowledge a problem. As a society we are so consumed with activity that we have lost our keen senses: vision, sight, and hearing, all imperative to making good intuitive decisions." I went on to explain how this applied to me. "I get fixated on the present moment. I feel that I just don't listen to my heart, my gut, and sometimes even God. As a result, the lessons become harsher. I simply need to awaken my instincts and listen. It is very much like the Verizon telephone commercials where you walk around with a network of support systems, but sometimes it takes God to halt you in your tracks as if to say, 'Can you hear me now'?"

Reflection:

In life, I have learned many lessons of differing intensity that sometimes pushed me to what I felt was the brink of my destruction. There are times when writing this book that I was able to see similarities in lessons that I thought I had learned, but in retrospect when adversity reared its ugly head, I struggled to put the lesson to use. I once became angry at myself for not being a quicker learner or better at applying skills thinking that God must get disappointed or impatient with me. Now as I sit back, I am sometimes thankful that the lessons had been difficult to realize because I have been forced to take a good hard look at myself. In the darkest of moments as a patient in the hospital I found there was always a ray of hope, a gentle soul, or a calm presence to be discovered. I am thankful for the hospital staff and patients who, on a daily basis, gave of themselves, helping me to ease my pain and find my way.

I believe it is true that things that are worth having are worth fighting for. If your life has you drowning and deprived of oxygen, it is imperative to fight with everything you have to overcome it. By taking that "lifesaving breath" you learn to appreciate the gifts you are blessed with and what the miracles inside of you can accomplish

POTHOLES

Each of us may be sure that if God sends us on stony paths He will provide us with strong shoes, and He will not send us out on any journey for which he does not equip us well.

Alexander Mac Laren

Chapter 9
The Unexpecting Heart Beats Normally

The heart beating is a natural, automatic occurrence we rarely think about. It functions without any effort from us, not requiring any input, yet it is critical to life. If it isn't working, neither is anything else. It responds to its environment simply taking only what it needs to survive and changes its rate accordingly counting every second of your life, like a fine watch.

Symbolically, the heart represents love–a basic need that can flourish if we allow it to or wilt and die if neglected. Love is nourishment for the body and soul. There are many levels, layers, and circumstances of love. It evolves with each type, whether for the joy of children, the comfort in a friendship, or the depth of a family member. It can explode into the lightening and luster of true romance. Love can be lazy like a vacation to the New England shore or as turbulent as the Bering Sea in midwinter. All types of love help the soul to evolve. Loss of love: any of the loves in life is difficult, if not impossible to overcome. I believe the greatest gift God has given us is the ability to love, but a broken heart can be devastating or even fatal.

Stability comes in many forms, dating Ray was mine. He was unthreatening and comfortable. We had a mutual agreement. We would see each other weekly to catch a movie, we'd look for each other when we could, and we talked daily on the phone for fifteen minutes at 9 p.m. It was a pattern that provided consistency, something I needed. It required very little time and effort for Ray and my part as well, so it worked. I had a date for every weekend, every dance, and no longer had to deal with the teenage "stalkers" that wanted to touch me. It was predictable and for the first time Roberta my beautiful stepsister, did not feel like a threat.

I was comforted knowing that my Ray who had once been interested in Roberta, now felt she was stuck-up and inapproachable. He couldn't have said anything greater to me. This confirmed to me that we were meant to be. We were the perfect pair, he was mine and I was his! Ray provided security and I was on top of the world. He was my knight in shining armor as his very presence defused the conflict in my life. He liked me and he was my first chosen sexual partner. He taught me what guys wanted and I was very eager to please, believing that if I kept him happy he would never leave me. I had the old belief that my "first love" would be the person I would marry. We dated all through high school.

When I was in tenth grade, Ray's dad became ill and soon after passed away. The loss was one I was too familiar with and I mourned right alongside his family. Ray's mother never recovered from her husband's death and Ray became the man of the house at fifteen-years-old. He had a difficult time handling it all, which brought us even closer together, as we bonded in our grief. I learned to hold on tightly; he, however, learned to be a player.

Young, wounded, and desperately wanting to move away from home, I moved in with Ray at 17-years-old. I was just too young to see at the time that Ray was not as committed as I was. I was repeating a pattern of choosing poorly.

Ray's mother, Mary Jane, seemed happy for the comfort of her son in her home, and I was happy to leave Wally behind. It wasn't just one thing that possessed me to come home from school one day and tell Wally I was moving out, it was a culmination of all of the ugliness through the years, things that I could not speak of, things people would not believe. I was tired of being abused and moving on seemed to be the answer; this was my escape.

I knew that if I could make Ray happy, I would have a forever home. Together, we could create a home where two people loved each other. Part of making him happy meant not forcing him to wear a condom. With the state of my self-esteem I had lost all insight into what was safe, and safe sex was not a practice I forced upon him. It was not in the manuscript of how to pleasure him. I could never bring myself to question him and believed he would take care of me. Needless to say, two healthy teenagers created new life.

I became pregnant at nineteen and decided to go through with the pregnancy even without Ray's support. I took a leave from college to plan for the baby and decided it would be best if we moved out on our own. Mary Jane was livid and rejected us from her life. "If my house isn't good for your family, then I don't want you here either," she would tell us.

I knew she was hurting to lose her youngest son and be left alone. If I had been at all stronger, I may have realized that we were not at all ready, seen the red flags and perhaps recognized she knew better than I. When I was eight-months pregnant I told Ray that if I were to raise this baby alone, she would take my maiden name. Yet, it was his mother who somehow convinced him "to do the right thing," which I guess was to marry me.

I believed in that silly fairy tale, that shiny ring impaired all my common sense, and I truly believed in happily ever after. I gleefully married Ray in March of 1984.

We had a nice little ceremony with a Justice of the Peace in our apartment surrounded by friends, separated from adult family whom didn't support our decision including Aunt Rita. We completed our vows and the usual rituals with my sister Joyce by my side.

When it was time to "kiss the bride," Ray not only kissed me but gave me a great big hug. We were in love and thought we were ready to take the necessary steps.

Despite our vows, Ray continued his usual nights out with friends. I remained at home, peaceful with the little life within me. I didn't impose on Ray to attend appointments or stress tests trying not to be a nagging wife. As my belly stretched to its fullest capacity I would lie in bed and lean up against him for comfort. As Amanda would roll or kick I'd hear, "Could you move away from me, I don't like the way it feels." I'd comply confused; unable to understand him

My delivery date came and went as my body grew increasingly uncomfortable and cumbersome. Dr. Loehfelm, my gynecologist decided to order a stress test to determine if inducing labor would be a safe option. Alone I went for the test and alone I returned home. The contractions continued however for almost forty-eight hours, and Ray grew impatient with me. I was exhausted and wanted to rest; I smiled as Ray went out with his friend Dominic. I went into active labor while Ray went into a drunken stupor. I waited at home while the contractions gripped me with pain and held their intensity for longer and longer. When Ray finally arrived home to take me to the hospital, I felt that I did not have any other options but to trust him to drive. The contractions were too strong, as so was my will to make things right for this new baby. The delivery experience inscripted what my life was meant to be.

My pains continued on through the night while I listened to Ray vomit from his once again too frequent, overindulgence in alcohol. His retching seemed almost as rhythmic as the contractions. I endured the pain as quietly as I could be cautious not to wake him. I had given up on him. I knew I needed to do this one on my own and as effectively as possible to self-preserve again. I put myself in my "protective bubble" and did what I needed to do. The sad thing was, I was glad to have him there. Still, I knew I needed to do this parent thing on my own. The self-preserve was again turned on and the "forward button" engaged. I would do whatever it took to make sure this baby was provided for. In my mind the choice I made was "till death do us part." The only thing that would force me to leave him would be infidelity. For now, it would be the three of us, forever. I would make things right for all of us.

As a baby Amanda was wonderful. She slept almost all night from the day I brought her home. Her dark, olive skin brought out her incredible dark brown eyes and thick, curly lashes. We nicknamed her "Amanda Roo." When she'd cry, he soothed her by singing her a song with that nickname in it.

"There was a little baby and her name was Manda Roo, Manda Roo," he sang.

I think it helped me to calm more than her. From the moment Amanda was born, my life had been filled with more love than I could have imagined, and we were both in love with Ray.

I didn't need anything from him, just his love. He worked, brought in money, and went out with his friends. I did not want to make him feel trapped. I hoped that eventually he would come around, and he did. He came around just long enough for me to become pregnant again. I was happy: he was furious.

"You are trapping me," he said.

I couldn't understand what he was implying. We were a family building a life. I loved being a mom and found the unconditional love gratifying. Ray, the man who refused to wear condoms wanted to know how this happened. Still, I believed everything would work out for us.

With a new baby on the way, we bought our first house, a sign that dreams can come true.

It was during my pregnancy that Wally was diagnosed with bone cancer. Despite all the pain I had endured because of him, I believed no one should suffer so severely. He fought for his life valiantly, yet multiple surgeries, resections, therapies, and even amputations could not subdue his aggressive killer. I'm not sure who suffered worse pain, me as a child or him in his death, but I would never wish either upon any living soul. Watching Wally through his struggle, I learned there were many paths to death.

Our daughter Erin never met Wally and she came into life with the urgency that marked her character.

I awoke from a sound sleep with a horrible thud. "Wham!" It felt like I had been punched in the stomach. It was dark and almost five o'clock in the morning. I rolled quietly trying not to disturb Ray and brought myself to my feet, still short of breath from the pain. "Whoosh!" My water had broken splattering on myself and the floor with full force. I immediately went into hard labor. I woke Ray pleading with him, "Ray, I need to go to the hospital now. The baby is coming."

The contractions had me doubled over with every task I attempted to complete, which made it a slow process to get out the door and into the car. As hurriedly as I could manage, we headed to the hospital with each bump in the road gripping me with pain. I walked to the front door as he parked the car fearing there was just no time.

I panted and struggled in the labor room trying to get my clothes off and to get on the labor room bed. It was there that Erin was born just before 8 a.m. that February morning in 1986. We didn't make it into the delivery room,

She had beautiful fair skin and mint green eyes. Her lashes and fuzzy hair were definitely going to be blonde like her father's. As a baby Erin was demanding, which made having two babies difficult for me. She cried or I should say screamed when she had a need and was very impatient. She seemed to know just how to get attention and was so cute people delighted in spoiling her.

We nick-named her "Erie Berry," pronounced (air-ee bear-ee). I had the help of my sisters and my mother-in-law Mary Jane, who at that point had been very good to me. It amazed me how babies bring families together. Life was difficult but filled with love. I had the dream that I wanted, mixed with all the realities of life. We now had the perfect little world, the so-called "American dream." I was very happy with my family and found complete happiness being a mom.

Ray continued life as usual and I continued making excuses for him. As the next years passed, our relationship became a little rocky. I tried not to challenge him. I wished for him to find the same happiness in our girls that I did and hoped he'd find a reason on his own to be with us. When he did come around, he took full advantage of my need to please him. It wasn't long before I became pregnant with our third child. I was thrilled, but he was very angry. He blatantly told me, "Three is too many. We can't have this one." He wanted me to terminate the pregnancy. I vehemently refused. Later, I found out it was a boy, my son Adam. For whatever reason, I felt that this would be the magic key to Ray wanting to be a member of this family. I was wrong.

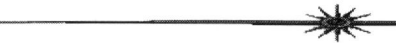

My third pregnancy and delivery were uneventful. When Adam was born in the spring of 1988 he looked like a little Indian baby. He had an eye color that was dark and indiscernible which later turned to hazel. He had thick, dark eyelashes and had round, full features. As a baby he was perfectly content, gentle, and calm. He just seemed to observe his world, requiring very little from me. I adored him. I had three uniquely beautiful children, more than anyone could ask for and I basked in the love that surrounded me.

Ray continued to be a good provider; he just did not know how to be a good father. I will be forever grateful to him for providing us with the stability that allowed me to grow. Ray was my first love, my first husband and the father of my children. Still, I knew that he loved his freedom more than the family life. He was well-loved by all, including me. We had everything, yet he did not know it.

He was a beautiful man, distinguished with blonde, thick, curly hair when we met, now shaved clean to disguise his receding hairline. None the less, he had an alluring presence and playful blue eyes with color that flickered with his changing moods. In those eyes I could see his soul, his love, and his hatred. He had a thick, rugged upper body and a downward curve to his shoulders that created a cradle in his arms when he held me. When he kissed me, the heat of his lips made me forget any troubles. That was one of my favorite things about him. I was so jealous of the definition of his body, something he maintained with minimal effort. He didn't spend hours in the gym to look great in a pair of jeans. To those that knew him, he was engaging, especially after a few beers at the bar, his second home. My friend Tracie called him "hottie butt," and it was true.

Our pattern took on the image of many dysfunctional homes. I stayed home to give my children the childhood I was deprived of. Ray went out with his friends after work. I never disturbed his life with his friends in fear that if I made any demands on him, he would leave me, or worse yet I feared the abusive drunk I witnessed so long ago. I held steadfast to my wish that Ray would wholeheartedly find happiness at home, but deep inside I knew he was already gone.

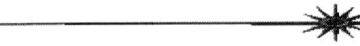

When Adam started kindergarten, I decided to go back to school to finish the education I had set aside to start my family. My dream was to become a nurse.

"I don't care what you do as long as it doesn't impact my lifestyle," he said.

Ray made it clear that my education was my choice not his. Without his support, I knew I had to push forward and become more independent. It was a difficult few years tending to the children before and after school then staying up all hours of the night to study while they peacefully slept. I was willing to sacrifice myself for our future, for all of us. The kids were too young to understand anything more than the fact that I would put them to bed at 8 o'clock and tell them from that point I was done being a mom for the day and needed to study. They still remind me of this.

My first nursing job as an RN was a shift working nights on a medical teaching floor. I loved it, and was on top of the world. I had completed my education and landed a great job working nights, three 12-hour shifts. It seemed least disruptive to our lives.

Ray seemed somehow threatened by my self-confidence and the salary I was earning just three days a week.

"A wife shouldn't earn more than her spouse, it's just not right Lin," he would protest.

"Lin" was a nickname he used when he was being curt with me. I knew we had a problem and I didn't know how to console his ego. I wanted to believe I was finally realizing my dreams and it would be a good thing for our family. I worked so hard, always hoping that all the good things would make that golden difference.

Ray made working increasingly difficult for me. He continued to stay out with friends even when I had to work. I would be panicked waiting for him to return so that I could leave, and feared losing my job. Often I relied on his mom, giving her short notice, to come watch the children.

Then one night I was called off from work due to a low census at the hospital. I was delighted to be home with my family. While we slept, the phone rang, and a truth I fought so hard to ignore broke through the silence of the darkness. Ray took the call and went deep into the house as he spoke. The call came at 1 o'clock in the morning on a night that I would normally have worked. Slowly, I put it all together and decided to follow him, pretending to be concerned that something had happened.

He abruptly ended the conversation when I approached. My heart was given a new glimmer of hope, a flutter. He did not want me to find out. I found consolation thinking he might still love me, still want me even though our bed was now empty.

"Is everything alright?" I asked trying to continue the expression of being genuinely concerned.

He lied. "It was a friend that just needed to talk," he nonchalantly said walking away.

I paused to process the information, yet perplexed. I asked, "What friend would call at this hour?"

He responded angrily, turning away, "I am going back to bed!"

Our bed, our sacred bed, I thought. I had grown accustomed to his anger being directed at me and my basic needs being brushed aside.

I stood alone briefly, cold in the kitchen, reduced to feeling like a berated child. Despite the luxury of being wrapped in a warm, comforting robe, it could not protect me from the painstaking truth. With anger overtaking me and blood flushing into my ears I pursued him into the bedroom. I picked up the phone and dialed *69 (then a new feature on the phone). I was shocked when a young female voice answered, confirming the whisper my heart tried to tell me and the truth my brain flatly denied.

She said, "Hello."

The Unexpecting Heart Beats Normally

"Hi, who's this?" I asked politely. I did not have to ask who she was, I knew her voice. I simply hung up clinging to the hollow ache in my heart that signaled my stomach to wretch and throw up. Immediately the phone rang again and I hung it up without answering it. It continued to ring and each time I hung it up without answering. Finally I looked at Ray and asked for the truth; he confirmed the name I knew so well.

Kim was a mutual "friend" who I assisted when she needed a job. She was young, perky, and energetic. She had a beautiful smile, engaging dimples, and baby doll eyes. I believed she had great potential–never knowing that while introducing her to a new job where my husband and I worked, I would be introducing my destructive fate.

The knife twisted in my chest creating a space for betrayal. My years of dreaming about happily ever after, believing that he would come around, were trampled. I never knew his intentions: for when I was dreaming of him, he was dreaming of her. I did not know how this could be. I believed I had done everything I knew to be right. I was a good mom, a good housekeeper, and a good wife that never refused him of anything. There was a whisper inside me, a yearning pride that pushed me to leave. I always promised myself that despite my burning loneliness, the lack of attention, and the verbal abuse, I would only leave for one reason; infidelity–and here it was. At this very moment my heart had been carved out and I left to die.

The one value I thought I could preserve now vanished. I felt disgraced and humiliated, but worse than that, became disappointed in myself as I was unable to be true to myself. Broken and disheartened, I decided to stay with Ray for the sake of protecting the stable lives of our three beautiful babies who didn't deserve this and needed their family. I fought to hide the piercing sadness through each day. I simply moved on.

For Ray's thirtieth birthday, I decided to throw a surprise party for him. I invited his entire family, my family, all the neighbors, and all his friends. The plans were complete with rented chairs, tables, a tent, catered food, and a full bar. I was so engaged in making this day a special event, nothing mattered. Everyone secretly panned to arrive at our home before he returned from work shortly after five on a Friday. We waited patiently visiting among one another anticipating his arrival which was much delayed.

When he arrived and everyone yelled, "Surprise!" Ray's eyes immediately searched the crowd to find me. I was ecstatic! I had pulled it off and my smile beamed from ear to ear. Ray, on the other hand, marched purposely toward me and scolded me for assuming he would be home on his birthday.

He told me, "I made plans and I am going out!"

I stood briefly, silently crushed, and then shook it off as I always did. I pretended that no one would notice and went on as if nothing happened. I knew whom he was choosing to spend his birthday with and he did. To this day I never asked anyone what their impression was of the whole thing. It was too painful and by now I had grown used to ignoring my pain.

I had become numb over the years and my complacency continued to grow. I stayed in the marriage, despite being humiliated and despite knowing who he was with when he didn't come home. Everyone around us knew the truth.

For many years I lived this lie pretending that Ray was faithful and we were a happy couple, a secret I thought was shared just between us. It wasn't until my children were adults that they confided in me they knew differently.

Amanda would inform me that she held his secret for many years. "Mom, I was so afraid to tell you, so afraid to hurt you." I learned that Ray shared my bed with Kim on the nights when I worked. The kids would hear her in the house while they pretended to sleep, too afraid to make their presence known, far too young to be expected to hold a secret of betrayal.

At her young eight years of age, an innocent and beautiful heart was left to carry the burden of guilt. Amanda's father should have protected her. She should have been able to trust him. Instead, she carried his secret knowing such a violation could destroy me. The fact is the destruction reached further than Ray cared to give thought to at the time, this burden etched in Amanda's soul was another trigger to her decline. I wished I could have erased these memories from my precious child's mind.

I found myself in an uncompromising situation: I was forced to forgive the unforgivable for the sake of my family. I had chosen this man, chosen to have children with him, and chosen to make a life with him. Reality was that my children did not ask to be brought into this situation and I needed to make it work for them. It didn't matter to me if I was happy, it only mattered that they had a stable environment to spend their remaining years in our home together.

I knew in the past that I was able to create a nurturing and loving environment void of their father's intercession, and I was determined to continue to do so. There would be a happier time for me later. I was willing to sacrifice. I still believed the unthinkable, that maybe with a few changes, Ray would have a change of heart (maybe I was at fault). I believed he was my soul mate. For this season of my life, I learned to love, learned to endure.

Reflection:

One of the greatest things in life that we can do for ourselves is to learn to love ourselves, our God, and to self-preserve. Love is truly a gift that has great potential. I believe true love can come from many levels and is not a perfect entity. In fact, love is often difficult to recognize or sort from other emotions. Each lesson occurs at the perfect place in time for us so that we might continue to evolve as individuals. I have found that each lesson has a spiritual purpose which allows us to grow into new relationships and enjoy different types of love. I am thankful for the ability to be able to experience this pure emotion. To me the opportunity for love is worth having and worth working for, but the greater gift is to know when it is time to move on.

In general, it is unrealistic to believe that we will or have to get it right in our lifetime, or even that the experiences of others will have the same outcomes as ours. Love can be a beautiful blessing, be taken for granted, or difficult to figure out until you've jeopardized it or lost it. The only consolation for me was the knowledge that I was working on myself within my relationship with Ray. I am thankful for the place he had in my life and the lessons I've learned because of him. I realize he was a perfect fit in a time when I could've spiraled out of control. With Ray I learned to love and to feel emotions! We made three beautiful children, and created a wonderful home. Together we took a journey that renewed my faith and you can't ask for more than that.

"When you and I hurt deeply, what we really need is not an explanation from God but a revelation of God. We need to see how great God is: we need to recover our lost perspective on life. Things get out of proportion when we are suffering, and it takes a vision of something bigger than ourselves to get life's dimensions adjusted again."

Warren W. Wiersbe

A Heart in Trouble Letting Go:

When vessels in the heart become narrowed and stiff, the heart muscle works exceedingly hard to force blood through constricted or entirely occluded areas, often with little or no success. As a result, the heart gets fatigued from excessive exertion and cannot be nourished properly. Prolonged, the insufficient blood flow may cause a portion of the muscle to die; bypass surgery using veins from the lower body may be an option to provide an alternate path for blood to flow.

When the veins are harvested they are "stripped" of the valves within them, which make them more suited to create free circulation; readily supplying the heart with the nutrients it needs. Its effects are noticed almost immediately and the patient's overall quality of life may be renewed.

Although there were many events in my life that could have led to my demise, I believe the culmination of many things contributed just as they do in heart disease. For me, the healing process began with forgiveness, letting go, and blind faith.

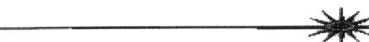

My sister and her new boyfriend Mark had come to see me in the hospital. Joyce was still not divorced; in fact she left Daniel absconding to Florida with her kids and the over $60,000 she indeed removed from Daniel's bank accounts. I worried for her safety and mine. It was there that she met Mark and without hesitation rented a home and moved in together.

I found it a peculiar fate that she and my daughter Erin were literally neighbors now after all the events that had occurred, but there was relief knowing neither of them was alone.

I tried to not focus on the loss I felt when Erin left, or the anger I felt blaming Joyce that my life had spontaneously combusted. Those wounds still hurt, I had forgiven, but trust was tough to recover, and I couldn't forget.

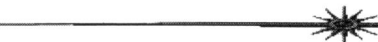

I thought it was a selfless gesture on Joyce's part to drive out to see me with Mark. They spent a portion of the day in my room. Mark worked overnights so he slept on the sofa allowing Joyce and I some quality bonding time. She had been thoughtful enough to bring some familiar things from home. I know it had to be difficult to see her big sister this way, especially since we had once been so close, and since Patti had lost her battle to the same disease, and for the time we lost. I understood her insecurities or at least I tried.

When Joyce was stressed she tended to babble or busy herself with little things that needed to be done. In watching her I realized that she struggled with the same inability to relax as I did. She got up to re-stuff Bessie. She tried to busy herself attending to me but eventually her impulsivity won. She blurted out, "This is boring! How can you stand it?"

I paused a moment after hearing the frustration and helplessness in her voice. I thought, *Here I am tethered to my bed, feeling helpless, and she is bored*? I searched myself trying to find an appropriate response. I took a breath, looked her in the eyes and replied, "I know, I have been here a long time, almost sixty days, watching as the world goes by, but I have been blessed with the opportunity to focus on myself, doing absolutely nothing, and preserving my energy for now so that I may live long enough to be blessed with an organ."

I believe the visit was peaceful and healing for the both of us. When she left, I experienced an incredible let down, both missing her when she had gone, and mourning all of the years we had lost. She always touched my heart, which had simply allowed me to let my guard down; it was painfully beautiful.

I wasn't allowed much time to wallow in self-pity because I started to receive multiple phone calls and visits after she left. Somehow God continued giving what I needed. My cousin Michael and his wife Marsha called and cheered me up. Mike has a great sense of humor. "Why don't you just eat that bunny?" he joked. "You'll feel better," he continued.

He and Marsha had a wonderful, loving marriage, and a deep spirituality that I admired. Somehow the two of them complimented one another and simply found joy in life's little pleasures; including each other. As jovial as the conversation was, I don't think they believed there was sincerity in my voice when I asked him to bake a cake and put a nail file in it!

I got a visit from Julie the new patient on the floor. She was younger than I with small children and wasn't a candidate to remain in the hospital. She was a difficult cardiac match because of immunity factors and her high priority. She stayed at home waiting and was admitted intermittently when her heart was in crisis. We talked quite awhile and she headed on her way. Somehow I sensed something more needed to be said.

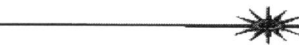

My former neighbor Joan also called then. I was thrilled to hear from her. She had been battling leukemia and her voice wavered as she spoke, yet it uplifted me knowing I had another lifeline. We began to reminisce on a past I had tucked away many years ago. She knew all my secrets with Ray. I was good friends with her, and adored her daughter Barbara and granddaughter Leah, who was the same age as my daughter Amanda.

Barbara died suddenly after a fatal asthma attack. It was the closest loss to me since the death of my sister. Ironically, Barb was on life-support and declared "brain-dead" too –just like Patti. As painful as it was to relive Patti's death, that experience enabled me to support Joan through the process of "pulling the plug" too. Barbara was forty-one and one of the most vibrant, happy, and energetic people I had ever known. Her smile and laugh were contagious. Once again a life lesson had repeated itself. Everything happens I believe so that you can help someone else. Though Barb's family felt great sadness by her death, they brought other families great joy with the gifts of her organs.

The walk down memory lane with Joan was quite therapeutic.

I continued to receive e-mails that day from people in prayer chains all over the world. It was quite impressive to see so many people come together for a common purpose: and it was me! My room became a sanctuary and I began to notice a restorative balance in my life. I was content, grateful, and comfortable.

Later that day, Kristyn came by and we talked about the change in me. She asked what had occurred.

"My entire life, all this time I was fighting to keep some sort of control because it was what I knew. I had always had to fight for my place in life and I didn't know how to let go. The only thing in my life I could equate to losing that level of freedom and giving in was a prison sentence," I told her.

She looked at me oddly.

I continued, "I had recently watched the movie, *Shaw Shank Redemption*, and while I watched, all I could think about was how powerless prisoners were. I saw a parallel in my hospital stay. I was confined to my room with a commode in the corner. Being a prisoner was the only parallel I could find to giving up control and moving forward," I told her.

Kristyn simply smiled and listened.

The nurses had begun shutting my door during the day to allow me to rest. It was probably a good thing, but it also made me feel isolated. I needed isolation; I was simply getting too sick to see visitors.

Chris always told me I gave to the point of self-destruction and I finally understood what he meant. I realized that I couldn't give in the way I had anymore. *Yes there is a fine line between giving of you and giving yourself away,* I thought. *I simply have nothing else to give right now.*

I know the analogy is a little harsh, but I have to be honest, it was my salvation. For the first time in my life, I was able to trust and let go without intervening when things didn't happen quickly enough. Amazingly, once I surrendered, good things began to happen. I felt safe and protected, happy and peaceful, and was filled with ease of mind and heart.

Reflection:

As my heart continued to fail, as I became increasingly exhausted, my capabilities lessened and I became dependent on others to recognize my weaknesses and advocate for me. I resisted at first, but soon realized that they knew best and it was alright to let it go. When I woke in the morning I acknowledged God in my life and asked Him, "O.K., you've given me another day, what would you like me to do with it?" When I closed my eyes at night, I viewed my life as a journal. With each page I took notes and studied hard. Life's lessons are the building blocks for your soul. I was not a victim, but the recipient of great lessons.

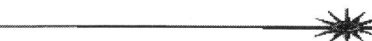

You cannot cure the soul of others or "help people" without having changed yourself...You cannot bring peace to others if you do not have it in yourself.

Alexander Elchaninov

POTHOLES

Chapter 10
Roo's Broken Heart-When a Policy is Bad Practice

The overall function of the heart occurs because of an intricate electrical conduction system. Each chemical works in sync with the brain and body ensuring absolutely flawless delivery. Amazingly, there are no wire, nor switches, just impulses that inherently know exactly what to do. When the heart is defective as was mine, the perfect balance is destroyed and like a bomb it ticks with a potentially fatal outcome.

The term cardiomyopathy refers to weakening of the heart muscle and failure refers to changes and symptoms that occur because of it. When medical science was able to identify that I indeed had the genetic marker for a type of cardiomyopathy, it was like a life sentence had been handed down. Through most of my life I knew there was a connection to the suspicious deaths of so many family members, but no one understood who it would affect, when, or why.

Maybe I was in denial, but I did everything I believed was right to take care of my heart so that it didn't have to happen to me. I wanted to be the first survivor, instead of another statistic.

POTHOLES

My condition was the result of a genetic mutation, called "phospholamban." In some way, I was ecstatic to be a part of the study published in Science magazine back in 2003, but it is bittersweet to have the "disease" now defined. It was explained to me that as a result of this mutation, calcium is not able to be used properly in my heart's electrical system. It is an amazing concept that one simple deficit can lead to a series of potentially terminal events. Just like in life mistakes happen, some we can prevent, some we can prolong, some we are helpless to do anything about.

Amanda was a jovial child. She was the perfect little princess and typified by the "first-born." She spoke articulately and aimed to please by modeling grown-up behavior. She loved wearing her pretty dresses with her patent leather shoes and her hair neatly combed into pig tails. She reminded me of "Cindy Lou Who" in Dr. Seuss' "The Grinch Who Stole Christmas." She was polite and soft spoken–almost melodic.

Amanda had a knack for self-entertaining or helping around the house and could occupy herself for hours at a time. She loved to vacuum and even wash the dishes. She developed wonderful friends among her toys and was a great little mommy.

As long as her needs were met, she was happy. Even as an infant, I could see the love in her playful brown eyes as she nursed and watched my every move. She was rarely demanding. She loved when we read bedtimes stories, her favorites included a series called "Teach Me About." The book on potty training made her giggle. Her face would light up as I changed my voice for each character in the book. I was proud that she was my daughter and loved my "little companion." She had many favorite toys and took good care of them by lining them up on her bed.

Amanda also had a great deal of respect and love to offer animals of all types. She would bring home any stray animals she saw including "Fleagers" the cat that was in fact infested with fleas.

She had a bunny named Carmel that we used to keep on a leash in the yard. Once, Carmel got her paw caught in the leash and began to cry an eerie scream. Yes bunnies scream when they are terrified. Amanda ran to her bunny to save her from the danger, but that sound was one she did not soon forget.

A few years later while working in the yard, we both heard a similar cry. She began to look through the high grass for the origin. As I started out walking over to Amanda to help her she began to scream.

"MOOOOOM help!" she cried.

Running now, I got there in time to see a snake eating a frog. I tried to rationalize with her that it was part of nature, but she pleaded with me.

"You have to save it mom, you have to," she pleaded convinced I could "fix it."

I was afraid of snakes, but picked up a stick and swatted the snake on the head. The snake lurched backward dropping the frog, and seemed to look at me confused by what had happened. The frog on the other hand, was my main concern. Although stunned momentarily, it soon began to hop away. By then, the snake was long gone.

I envisioned if the snake could speak what it would say. I imagined a scenario: "Ouch! What are you doing lady? That was my dinner!"

Amanda was so grateful; I felt like a hero. I'm not sure how many moms would have done the same, yet we all have pivotal times in our lives when we recognize the depth of what a mother's love can be.

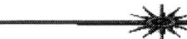

At around the age of seven Amanda had repeated throat infections and required a tonsil and adenoidectomy. The next few years following the surgery lacked a normal recovery. She began to gain weight at an alarming rate; fifteen pounds in the first year alone, and I became concerned. On occasion she would lose consciousness for brief seconds that seemed an eternity. Her eyes simply rolled back into her head and her body became lifeless. The doctors tested her and only concluded that her body was overcompensating for her weakened health prior to surgery. I didn't realize then, she was harboring the truth about her father.

Looking back, I realize that balance, harmony, and life circumstances impact your health. Amanda was not healthy. She held in an invisible "cancer" that was beginning to grow at her young age. It was a disease that I hadn't realized that I helped plant and didn't know how to prevent. I had missed that glaring moment to help heal Amanda and change her life's course; instead, I lived in denial. My marital bed was shared with another woman. When I left for work, she came in. Amanda's little heart held a secret that grew like cancer. My denial of the situation grew out of a need for security. I wanted the perfect home; but did not know how to create it. There was just so much I didn't know then.

As Amanda grew older, she became rebellious and more difficult to communicate with. She began to dye her hair with Kool-Aid, at first single colors and later rainbows of color. As a parent, I decided to allow her to express herself seeing these acts as harmless. Occasionally I played parent and threw in a comment about my displeasure. I did not have the confidence to take charge; to be the strong parent. I was caught in a society that promoted uniqueness and creativity. I wanted to be the best parent for my child in a world that was telling me to allow her to express her uniqueness – to pick my battles. Yet in Amanda I perceived a hole in the center of her young heart. It called out to me to protect her from invisible dangers. I realized that I could have allowed her creative to flourish in the art room, instead of her hair. The fact was, she was troubled, she needed me, and I simply failed to listen to my inner core.

I did not prod her to stay on the path of peaceful stability as I should have, in retrospect. Then, I did not have the wisdom to see the truth. She needed clarification, not confusion. She needed a solid foundation.

One of her most impressive hair colors was teal! As her efforts became more intense, so did her cries for help. I missed them entirely. One day, I took her out shopping with that awful color and I told her she looked like a "Smurf!" In the store, a customer told her the color was beautiful. As a parent I was confused, it was not beautiful, in my opinion it was ridiculous. It seemed the more dramatic the effort, the less I gave her in return and in that brief encounter I took a second look at my daughter through someone else's eyes. Not only was the color beautiful, but so was my daughter. I had just gotten stuck in the pattern of destruction that was being set. Amanda did not need to be flamboyant; she needed stability and unconditional love.

I was not given the tools to be an effective parent and out of my confusion, destruction grew. I did know that I loved Amanda and I would fight for her, but I simply did not know what to do. She was setting the stage, making the rules, and I was losing control; something that I did not even see at the time. The invisible force was silently creeping into my house; taking over.

As she progressed into a teenager, she upped the ante. She became angry and irrational. Fear crept into my veins as I no longer recognized her. Amanda was no longer the beautiful little girl I once knew. Her anger had turned into rage and I was even afraid for my life. I half-joked among my friends about whether "I should sleep with one eye open." Again, I was a fearful child yet in the safety of my own home. The pattern I had fought so hard to leave had returned again through my flesh and blood.

Amanda's first boyfriend Josh was tall and gangly with dark green eyes and a deep voice. Amanda seemed to surround herself with him at every opportunity, yet their relationship appeared off balance. Josh didn't appear to be quite as smitten with her. .

I shared some insights with Amanda about safe, healthy relationships and about always being in control. I wanted to educate her about self-respect, and not letting anyone or any substance get in the way of making a good decision. In retrospect, those words may have been the reason she didn't come forward when she was in trouble: fear of disappointing me.

Amanda had fallen in love with Josh and had many of the same morals that I did as a young teenager. It frightened me because I had made poor decisions then, and it appeared as though she may do the same. He was not good for her and treated her poorly, but she found great pleasure in their co-dependent relationship–as I had with Ray. She felt needed with Josh and chose him as her first sexual partner. She harbored many trust issues in male relationships because of her father's relationship. I began to notice her life was traveling down a parallel path to mine despite my efforts to protect her from that.

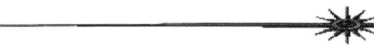

One night Amanda went to a party with a group of friends whom she hung out with frequently. I got a call from one of the parents asking me if Amanda could spend the night. I asked to speak to Amanda but was told she was upset about something that had happened at the party and would discuss it with me tomorrow. Tomorrow never came. Amanda spiraled downward after that. The ugliness had now taken root.

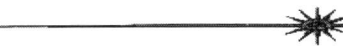

I tried valiantly to be there for her, but my timing never seemed right. My quality time became getting up in the morning with her and helping her to get ready for school, even though she was too old for me to do that now. We both needed the comfort. She would wake me to help her fix her hair at five-thirty in the morning. I noticed that her presence changed since the night of the sleep over. She always seemed panicked, pressured, irrational, but I could never get her to tell me the truth of that night, no matter how many times I combed her hair. I believed I should cherish the good moments since they were becoming so few and far between.

One morning when I was curling her hair she was talking about school when she paused mid-sentence.

She looked at me and said, "Mom, I feel like...." At that point her eyes rolled back in her head and she buckled into me.

I eased her to the floor and I could see she was pale and unresponsive. This time was different. I searched for a pulse, one I couldn't find, yet in my mind I was pleading with God for help. With the most blood curdling scream I called out, "Ray, call 911!" I couldn't bring myself to leave my baby on that bathroom floor all alone. I was terrified!

A flurry of thoughts ran through my head. *This can't be happening,* followed by, *I need to do CPR!* For a brief moment I sat back on my heels wanting to collapse into the floor beside her and cry. I thought, *This shouldn't be happening,* and the room spiraled around me. I thought, *I have never done CPR outside of the hospital without a medical team surrounding me–especially on someone I loved.* Suddenly, a voice from within called me to reason, "You have no choice!" I initiated CPR and with the first few breaths, my beautiful girl began to come around. After the ambulance arrived and I think I went into shock. My thoughts drifted back to the last time an ambulance had come... when my mom had died.

We rode to Children's Hospital where they performed a full evaluation, but they found nothing. I was told she had a sensitive central nervous system and that she should outgrow it. I had saved my child's life, yet I knew the truth. She still was not alive in spirit. The hospital could not heal her, she needed to heal herself; the war within her continued over the next few years. I tried to convince myself that these were typical teen "growing pains," but they were not. When you're too close to a situation, you can miss the clues. My daughter was having more difficulties than she cared to share with me, and all I knew was that I was there trying to save her life from becoming as ugly as mine. I was frightened for her and sought help through a program called PINS (Persons In Need of Supervision). It was a court appointed program for kids in trouble. Amanda was angrier than I had ever seen when the judge scolded her.

She looked at me stating, "You don't know what I am going through!"

She was right, but I didn't know what else to do. After that she seemed to pull the pieces of her life together.

As she entered her senior year of high school, she appeared to be committed to a better direction, with more focus–as if healing was beginning. Yes, there were many tear-filled nights, she couldn't handle the "block scheduling," it was too long to remain in class and stay focused. She admitted she had a problem, stating, "In my head."

I called the guidance counselor at the school on several occasions asking to refer Amanda for services. At that time, he felt, perhaps he would be able to address her personally. As those first few weeks progressed, she became increasingly emotional and refused to go to school, often sobbed hysterically. We had many tears over the September 11th incident, as Amanda reflected on the unsafe world she would be living in. She began to fear drinking the water, opening the mail, going to school: I thought the fears were due to terrorist attacks.

Terrorism was the excuse used to deny her real source of pain. The truth is terror was allowed into our house. We did not establish boundaries to prevent it. We embraced it, talked about it, and it allowed us to have something in common to discuss. We thought it united us, again allowing seeds of secrets to grow, destroy. We were victims and felt helpless.

I again approached the counselor. He referred her to the school psychologist which required the typical "referral process." I was getting impatient, but thought I saw a glimmer of hope when Amanda decided she'd like to go to the Homecoming Dance. We bought the gown and all that went with it; but she cautiously anticipated it. The underclassmen of Erin's class were working on a float at my home where Amanda helped with it.

One evening a group of students came in my yard to destroy the float, and Amanda was outraged that anyone would violate our property; her "safe" zone. After that incident, it took much prompting to get her to go to school again. I knew it would be a highly emotional day for her and my younger daughter, Erin. I called the school principal to notify him of the incident and asked him to intervene to avoid any altercation that could potentially occur. He assured me he would, but actually did nothing.

I received a phone call that day at 10:30 a.m. that Amanda had been suspended; the student approached her, and a shoving match occurred. Amanda was defending her sister Erin. I was told that due to school policy, Amanda would not be allowed to attend the Homecoming Dance because she had been involved in this incident! No one admitted to any wrong-doing for having not acted to protect my daughter as they were supposed to do; no one was there for her!

This resonated in my mind over and over. No wonder why she felt so unsafe! I was furious at this decision and spoke with several administrators that day, explaining suspension would be a poor choice of punishment; she hated school, was now humiliated, and was further banned from the first event she chose to participate in. I was told there would be other activities and the decision stood.

Amanda did not go back to school. She ended up being diagnosed with Panic/Anxiety disorder, underlying depression, and Post Traumatic Stress Syndrome. I initiated counseling, medication therapy, and home-teaching.

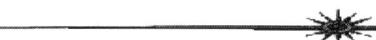

Desperate to get help for my daughter I took drastic steps. I faked an illness and went to my doctor as a "walk-in." There was nothing wrong with me but I needed help and felt no one was listening. They took my co-pay, weighed me, checked my vital signs, and the nurses did the basic assessment going through all the appropriate motions to bill the insurance company. I was determined to be heard, determined not to lose Amanda. I would not let the bureaucratic system deprive me.

When the doctor came in I began to sob, "Why does it take so much red tape to get help? Why did it have to come to this? I have tried all the expected channels to no avail and now my daughter's life had come to this." I confessed why I was there. The doctor wrote me an order for Paxil for Amanda, and referred her to therapy. I was silently relieved.

Through her counseling I learned of what nourished her "terror," and also the truth that she had been sexually assaulted by a student at that party so long ago, another secret. My feelings were churning, *I knew I should have gone to get her that night,* I thought, I blamed myself for not listening to my intuition. I believed she didn't tell me because I placed such high expectations on her by telling her to always be in control. My mind was scrambled.

"I was at the party with my friends and I must've passed out. I don't know what happened. I didn't drink a lot and we were having fun. I think someone put something in my drink. When I woke..." Amanda continued, sobbing, "he was above me! Where were my friends, mom? Why did they let this happen?" She couldn't continue and sank into the couch.

I sat beside her and the therapist finished the story.

"She was raped," the therapist told me.

Roo's Broken Heart - When a Policy is Bad Practice

I crumbled hearing her story, knowing that familiar pain. I had been unable to protect her. My daughter had been violated as had I.

She did not want to press charges as she couldn't bring herself to continue to relive the situation over and over. I wasn't sure what was best and followed the lead of the professionals. She just wanted to be assured that she would never have to face this student again. She could no longer endure the pain associated with attending the school where she would have to face her rapist along with the people she felt betrayed by. It took many months of rebuilding and tears to establish a safe environment for her, and years of continued recovery.

I had developed a "one day at a time" mentality and hoped to push her toward graduation. Amanda worked so hard through the trauma, adversity, changes, and healing. I was proud of her efforts. She had one course to complete in summer school due to a teacher conflict. The classroom teacher didn't feel the home-teacher was qualified to home-teach the course and refused to forward the information. The power struggle with the school system continued. *If they only had put half as much effort into the kids who needed them as they did into their shining stars*, I thought.

The Senior Prom approached and Erin was invited to attend, but Amanda did not express an interest to go until a few days later. She felt she needed closure with her friends. The prom was scheduled in a "safe" place, not the school. I called the school on Wednesday, not realizing ticket sales went off sale Tuesday. I left a message. On Friday, prom day, my call was returned. "We are sorry, Amanda cannot attend, Mrs. Brophy, ticket sales are over," I was told. Again this system remained inflexible and seemed to have no sense of compassion.

As a parent, I was outraged. As a human being working in the field of mental health and disabilities, I realized this decision could be very damaging. This was a giant step toward her recovery! I asked for a compromise.

"Can she buy her own dinner and join the dance later?" The answer was again no. Their decision was that she would only be allowed to attend the post-prom party at the school. The school that never supported her, the school system that didn't protect her, the building that housed her rapist! They made no attempts to consider this child as an individual.

I went upward to the Superintendent who stated, "She is not eligible to attend because the policy was that she had to be an actively participating student, attending school (not a home study student) in order to go to the prom." It was a new rule, another story, another source of despair.

I was a mother, fighting for her daughter. The system looked at her as a broken student; I looked at her and saw my baby fighting to survive. I fought back with everything I had in me. Something inside me called out for justice; this was larger than the prom. It was a path to make things normal for her. I lost all common sense and allowed her to pick a dress, a tux, the garter, and flowers to prepare for a change of heart. I believed there had to be some way, someone who cared to make a difference.

I made a few phone calls to local respectable community members. The decision stood, and I heard comments like: "If she's not well enough to go to school, she shouldn't be allowed to attend the prom," from school administrators.

After many failed negotiations, I decided to take her to the prom anyway. I just felt compelled to show her that she meant something; that she was worth the extra step, and she deserved better. I felt her rights were being violated and couldn't rest without doing something about it. The dress was a beautiful brown shimmering gown with spaghetti straps, and clear iridescent sequins. We complimented it with elegant gold jewelry and a wrist corsage. On her it was stunning and her olive skin glowed. We picked up Josh and I invited the local news. When we arrived, we were blocked from entering and I was reprimanded for showing up. The new excuse became no ticket, no entry. I even offered to buy them, but the answer remained firm.

We left in tears, I will be forever torn. My childhood had been so damaged and now my daughter suffered through hers. I wanted to fight for her because nobody did for me. As a child, I learned to fight, be in charge and take control. I wished now, I would have taught her peacefulness and harmony. We could have gone out to dinner at an expensive restaurant, just us. We would now have a memory of peacefulness. We could have talked about how the school tries to put methods into place for security. It would be a memory to look back on and make us smile, not cringe. The school system saw her as a risk, I thought of her as mine. I heard a small voice inside me, quietly saying, you will be okay. I knew I needed to take time to start listening to that little voice, that guidance from above. Calmness will replace fighting. It is a very effective tool.

Every student has the right to attend their prom; I still wished the situation could have been handled with a little compassion, even from me. She would never have another chance to go to her prom but if I could recreate that night for her, I would allow her to see a peaceful mother, not one that is fighting for her rights. I would be a mother with knowledge. It would be the knowledge that we would agree that there are rules and regulations in place that are necessary for us to live by. It is not about only us, we need to work for the good of the whole. Life is not fair and it never will be. How we respond to things that upset us create our world. I wish we could reflect back on that time and she could feel content. Instead, it may take years to repair the damage

Amanda made a comment that night that I will always remember. "Mom, they were never willing to help me," she told me.

To this day I know that I did try to help Amanda. I only wish my methods of fighting were replaced with creating. I wish I had created a positive memory to provide for a positive future. Yet, maybe my methods were seen for what they were intended for, to fight for my child to have a better life.

Soon after, Josh had a relationship with another female friend. Amanda, unlike me refused to tolerate it for any reason. She not only broke off with him, but called the new girlfriend to let her know he was seeing them both. It was one of the first times I saw her put her beliefs first. I was envious she had learned this and wished I had done the same.

To this day I am very proud of who my daughter is and how far she has come. She continued her counseling for many years and has been able to establish a loving relationship and two beautiful children. I believe those children saved her life, as did mine. She has a wonderful purpose and is the best mother you could ever wish for your grandchildren. Of course her life is not absent of challenges because just like you and I we all have lessons to learn and mistakes to make. I am glad that I have had the opportunity to make them right alongside her. Despite all the heartache and pain, she has become a wonderful young woman, an intellectual, confident and wonderful human being. In the face of adversity, it all works out. We just need to love one another and pick each other up when we fall.

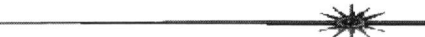

Reflection:

I don't believe I am defined by my past but I have taken my past as a means to define my future. My past is exactly that, the past, and it was an integral part of creating the person I am today. It is counterproductive to carry painful baggage, to place blame, and relive the ugly truth. It requires too much energy to allow negativity to thrive and creates a high level of anxiety which prevents us from growing.

POTHOLES

    Instead, I now acknowledge the role my past played, the emotions it stirred, and the reactions I had as simply a foundation for me to build on. It's not perfect and I still make mistakes, but I am alright with being the best person I know I can be.

Every adversity, every failure, every heartache carries with it the seed of equal or greater benefit.

Napoleon Hill

A Heart's New Life Flutters Within:

Heart failure is prevalent in millions of people in American and yet is poorly understood. It is the leading cause of human mortality and morbidity. On the molecular level, it is too complicated for me to understand. My heart failure is caused by a mutation. That may make me defective or maybe I am just special.

What I truly am, is a survivor, unwilling to accept that this is the way it is supposed to be. I believe I was born to be an opportunity for medical science to explode. I am at the forefront of miracles and am ecstatic to be a part of it! I have a priceless investment in the cure: my children and grandchildren.

I woke up to day sixty-seven in the hospital. There was a vase of lilies on my bedside table. They were from Julie; she had left them when she was discharged to go home. I was thrilled but envious she was home. I was tired of being in the hospital. My room was getting to be mundane, the bulk of my flowers had just about all died, and the routines were getting old. I had a line in my neck which meant the peer group was going to meet in my room at 1:30 p.m. Today I was the hostess.

I got myself cleaned up and was hanging out sitting in my bed. Dr. Nohria headed into my room with her usual routine. She smiled brightly, walked briskly, and acknowledged all of my personal things as she approached my bed.

It was the usual questions, "How are you, Any chest pain, shortness of breath or difficulties?" My answers were always no, but I was distracted because she had moved my water bottle from my bedside table to my nightstand. I couldn't reach it. As she talked, I thought, *Make sure she puts that water bottle back before she leaves.*

"Well," she said, "if that's the case, you can have nothing to eat or drink, I think we have a heart for you."

I was still fixated on the water bottle as she started to leave the room. Then it hit me.

"Wait! What does that mean?" I asked.

Pausing in her steps, she turned around smiling and returned to the bedside. "Right now we have a heart that looks like a good match. There are still some details that will need to be worked out," she told me.

"Should I call my family?" I asked.

"Yes," she replied.

For the first time in a very long time both my physical heart and emotional heart were beating as one. I was convinced God had a higher purpose for me and I was truly ecstatic!

After she left, I didn't know where to start; I wanted to cry tears of joy. I realized it was time! After all of the waiting, worrying, and preparing, my chance to continue in this life had arrived. I was thrilled and frightened all at the same time. I called Chris at work. "How would you like to come to Boston?" I asked.

There was a brief pause on the phone line. His disbelief and relief were both obvious.

"Really?", Chris asked.

I was so excited; I practically giggled a gigantic, "Yes!"

"I'll get there as soon as I can...I love you, see you soon." He hung up the phone long enough to make preparations for his journey to Boston and to notify our families. He called back to tell me that he was unable to get an immediate flight so he and his father decided the seven-hour drive would be faster, as did my children whom also chose to drive. I worried they might not make it in time, knowing a donated heart was only viable for a few hours outside the human body once harvested. Once things started in motion, it all goes by very quickly even though each minute seems endless.

Since I was a little nervous about being alone, I called my friend Loren to see if she could come stay with me. I was thrilled to hear she would as Loren had become invaluable now through this time in my life. Once Loren arrived we busied ourselves talking as we packed belongings from my room, both of us trying desperately to calm our nerves.

Many people within the team came in and out like a revolving door. There were consents, blood draws, surgical evaluations, and of course the ABC news team recording every aspect of my day. The nurses that had taken care of me during my stay stopped by randomly, Dr. Seideman, Dr. Stevenson, Kristyn, Katherine, Barbara, and all of the folks who had seen me through to this point. I was surrounded by earth angels.

My transplant friends, now only Lauren and Dr. Ken met in my room as a matter of routine that day. I was happy for me but worried about them. I wasn't allowed to let them know I had been called for a heart and that was grueling!

After the meeting was done, I made a few phone calls and left a few messages. One of those calls was to Stephanie. She was a transplant patient from Georgia and had connected with me previously. She wasn't home at the time, so I left a message about the big event and my gratitude for her presence in my life. Her returned call was the last call I received that day and her message was priceless.

In her beautiful, melodic voice I heard her say, "When they wheel you into the operating room, envision yourself being placed in God's hands, and let go. He will see you through."

This was exactly what I did and I was at peace.

I was unable to use my phone from that point forward because there was a problem with the carrier and I panicked knowing that people may try to reach me, including Chris. One of the nurses loaned me her phone for the day which acted as a safety net, but for those last hours I silently waited, I bonded with Loren and reflected quietly. I believed that God's plan for me at this time was to prepare myself peacefully, to put all else aside at the cusp of this moment. Having made the long journey to the hospital, my children, Chris, and his Dad arrived. It was a beautiful sight to see it all unfold. I couldn't have been more delighted that they were all there for me! I was surrounded by love and smothered with kisses. I believed then that God would take care of me.

I felt a certain peace as my family followed into the elevator and almost all the way to the operating room around 11:45 p.m. My son Adam handed me his Lance

Armstrong bracelet, as a token of his love. I could see the fear in his eyes. Love flooded my heart as I was prepped for surgery and said my goodbyes (for now). Around midnight in the operating room, the team looked at me.

"And now we wait for the surgeon, Dr. Couper to give us the go ahead to begin your sedation. He's verifying that the organ is viable," I was told.

I realized this was the point Dr. Ken had been denied his transplant due to the vegetation. *How awful to have gotten so close,* I remembered, *while I was moving forward, both he and Lauren were still waiting.*

I hadn't realized that the donor and another set of cameras were in the adjacent room. The phone rang and I heard, "It's a go!" That was my last memory with my old heart. It was May 7, 2009.

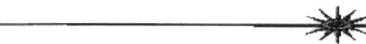

I had composed an e-mail to everyone I could think of to let them know what was going on and hit the send button before I headed to surgery. It read as follows:

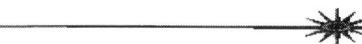

Hello Everyone,

This is the best possible way to let you all know that I was called for my heart transplant today. I kept this e-mail in draft form so that Chris would simply have to send it when the time came. There are so many things that I am thankful for: wonderful, dedicated friends, a very supportive loyal family, and the blessing of my faith. I feel very fortunate that I have had the time to adjust to being ill, and the incredible ability to compensate the way I have.

There are so many blessings. I can't thank any of you enough for the moments we've shared, and the impact you've had on my life. For now, it's time for the greatest gift a person can receive: the gift of life. Please pray for the best possible outcome…it's in God's hands.

*Love,
Linda*

For many the wait was unbearable and the potential for my loss very real. Strength is born in the deep silence of long-suffering hearts.

Felicia Hemans

Chapter 11
The Connected and Forgotten Hearts

When a heart is harvested from a donor, it is severed from the nerves and blood vessels that secured function in its body and then is transplanted into a foreign environment. Much like when a child is being born and the umbilical chord is cut, both need to adapt to their new surroundings in order to survive.

Once placed in the recipient's body, the vessels are grafted together and circulation finally will resume. These vessels are sutured and heal with minimal complication. In a person whose heart is intact the brain will tell the heart how to respond. For example, when a person exercises the body needs more oxygen and nutrients, so the brain will tell the heart to beat faster in order to meet the needs of the body. A donor heart, however, relies on circulating adrenaline in order to get it going. As a result, a heart transplant recipient must warm up thoroughly to get his or her heart pumping properly. The "denervated" heart can work almost as well as a normal heart. It's also possible for the donor heart to re-innervate–or grow nerves onto the donor heart.

In any crisis situation another type of disconnect occurs which is often not acknowledged. While the patient is the center of focus, the family members and the children are often left behind or assumed to be alright. The trauma they experience may in fact never be addressed causing *emotional troubles, responses, or health issues as life progresses.*

Survivor guilt surrounded me, and my psychological response to life experiences was atypical. Reflecting back, my heart still cried. The trauma I experienced may in fact never be addressed and may be the reason for some of my inappropriate emotional responses as an adult, or may have contributed to my health issues.

The loss of my parents and then my sister crippled my ability to have healthy, trusting relationships. I was afraid to get close to anyone, feeling they would not remain in my life; that they would leave by death or by choice. If I did learn to care or if someone told me that they cared, I found that I turned the other way or found a reason to end the relationship before it hurt me. In an effort to self-preserve or minimize what I couldn't accept, I denied and cowered. When I learned someone was ill, I was unable to be the supportive friend or devoted family member; I avoided the inevitable pain for as I long as I could.

I reminisce back to my Aunt Rita and how she dragged us to gravesites when we were young. In her mind, she was helping us pay tribute to those we loved and lost. What happened for me though was that I felt we were not able as children to create positive, loving connections to the living, but chronically being reminded of those that had left us behind.

Aunt Rita, my sister Joyce, and I were unable to adjust to life circumstances. There is not a map to guide a person through life or directions on how to be a perfect parent. It is even more difficult when the path is clouded by death and destruction.

My daughter Erin attracted much attention. She had the type "A" personality one might see with his or her first-born child, an over achiever and very competitive. She reminded me of my sister Roberta in that she was beautiful, confident, and self-directed. She walked by the time she was nine months old. Her thighs had triple rolls of baby fat that you'd never expect could bear her weight, but she was determined. With walking came potty training which she attained shortly thereafter. It seemed whatever her big sister could do, she mastered too.

Erin was methodical in everything; she lined up her toys often by color, type, or size, as well as her shoes, clothes, and other personal items. Everything had a place when she was young, as it should be. She was inquisitive and I often found her climbing into the garbage cans, the dryer, or just hiding waiting for someone to find her. She hated wearing clothes and her naked little body was usually covered with food or sand if she escaped to the sand box. Combing her curly, windblown hair was a challenge. I often chased her down and playfully sat on her so I could get the knots out. She still reminds me of that!

Her strong personality often clashed with Amanda's laid back style, and as children do, they often tangled. Erin would find refuge at the neighbor's house. Doug and Joan would always comfort her. They always kept a supply of treats for her and Erin always demanded one for each hand! She had a way of getting exactly what she wanted.

When Erin started kindergarten, the girls were playing in the yard swinging on willow tree branches when Erin's branch broke. Erin's arm had broken as well; snapping into a 90 degree angle. The school expressed some concern about Erin's ability to progress possibly needing to switch to writing with her left hand at this point in her education to keep from falling behind. To everyone's delight, Erin picked her pencil up with her casted arm and all, without hesitation. Nothing slowed her down.

She required minimal direction to do what was right and became actively involved in cheerleading, school activities, and friends. Like me, she buried herself in things to do to keep busy. Unlike me, she was loved endearingly by everyone.

She had strong commitment to her friends and chose relationships which could provide stability that I could not.

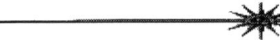

She found her main source of comfort in the unconditional love of Jason. He was full of compassion for life and was a volunteer fireman. He worked a few jobs at a time to put himself through school, and even worked alongside me with people with disabilities. His positive energy was abounding and his devotion unparalleled. They could be seen together almost everywhere. They loved to go out to eat and go to local events, especially at the fire hall. Erin loved chicken quesadillas and she could count on Jason any time to run out to get some for her literally day or night.

Jason also became a lifeguard which became an opportunity for them to spend long days at the local pools or beaches. She would bask in the sun while he'd remain perched in his stand protecting the lives of others. He was amazing and Erin had difficulty accepting how much he loved her at such a young age.

Erin worked for my sister Joyce as a waitress and tending bar at Ragoo's. She adored working alongside Joyce and their relationship grew daily. They shared common interests and both loved to be the center of attention in the "bar scene." She loved it all until she learned of the drug and alcohol that ran through people's veins; ruining their lives.

It was at this fragile age; Erin's world began to fall apart. Life as she knew it seemed to spontaneously combust; especially seeing her Uncle Daniel abusing not only drugs, but my sister Joyce, her aunt, first hand. Even more horrifying to her was the disappointment in her Aunt Joyce's drug use, and her failure to protect her children. Seeing her cousins Lauren and Perry thrust from their home into ours was more than she was willing to bear. A collision of two worlds made hers unsafe, and through this turmoil she was left home without a job. Shattered, bitter, and filled with hatred she ran away from everything. She did not want any ties; what she loved so dearly was a lie in her eyes, so she packed up and ran to Florida, leaving us all behind, including Jason in the hope for a new beginning.

Upon her first visit home for Christmas, Erin shared the news that she was going to have a baby. This didn't surprise me; it scared me. In an odd way, I understood it. She was repeating the same pattern, the same road map that I followed. She would leave her past behind, establish her own family in her own world, and she would do things right, even if she had started out all wrong. She would have this beautiful baby that loved her and she would master mommy hood. Things would be different. She did not see that she was isolating herself, denying that depression was creeping in.

We lay on my bed talking about her plans. Her main plan was to meet with Jason the next day, they had unfinished business and she wanted to be fair to him.

Unfortunately, she would never be able to speak all those words she had rehearsed so many times as her plans ended with a phone call. There had been in a terrible car accident. Jason had fallen asleep at the wheel. Erin called me at work to tell me the news sobbing uncontrollably. I met her at the hospital where Jason was in surgery for several hours while we waited with his family in the Trauma Center waiting room. Ken, Jason's dad asked us if we could clean Jason's his possessions out of his car for them. We agreed to fulfill their request and left to find the wreckage.

As we drove together, we talked about God's will and our beliefs. In this tragic and somber moment, a rainbow appeared. I remembered the Bible verse that the rainbow is God's promise to us that he will not destroy the world. I whispered to Erin that the rainbow resembled a ladder. I believed it was a sign. Her face went blank as she began to cry.

"No mom," she pleaded. We rode silently the rest of the way as I wrestled with God's plan and wondered if we had the strength to endure the hardships that continue to come our way.

Viewing the crushed vehicle, survival seemed impossible. The windshield, steering wheel, and seats were covered in blood, glass shattered along with our lives. We looked upon the wreckage in stunned silence; silence which was sharply broken when her phone rang. Jason's death was confirmed.

Erin burst into tears and we held each other for what seemed to be hours. Daylight came to a close and we finished our task in numb darkness. Jason had been a beautiful part of our lives for years. Watching his life end was darker than words can express. We attended his memorial as if he were our own family member, each moment engulfed in grief; doused in tears. The casket was closed draped with an American flag. Despite his short twenty-three years, Jason was honored as a hero. He was loved by many friends, coworkers, and was respected in the fire department. Outside the fire hall was his uniform, fire gear, and helmet: a tribute for the entire town to see. He was an angel in our lives.

I don't believe Erin recovered. She held great guilt about how their relationship ended; it lacked appropriate closure, and in his loss she realized that what she once had was what she truly desired but was too young to understand.

I added to Erin's pain by leaving her father. Erin was angry with me and blatantly asked, "What were you thinking?" I wrote her a letter that read as follows:

Dear Erin,

I think a better question is "What was I looking for?" I am very much like you. I am looking for someone to love me, to feel loved, feel secure, and to be able to count on someone. I want to be cared for unconditionally and I want someone to love all of my flaws. This in my world has always been my "fairytale," you know, the "Prince Charming" thing. I wasn't at all looking for it; I just believed it was out there.

When I enrolled at Houghton College, I had absolutely no goal; I just wanted the Bachelor's degree. I had no intention of leaving my job as CSDD, or leaving Dad at the time. To be honest, Chris was a student; I gave him minimal thought and not even a second look. My impression was that he was a nice dresser, neatly groomed, but basically a hot-headed man. I didn't sit near him nor talk to him at first. I learned personal things about him from speeches he made in the classroom, but really that was it. It was a Christian School. We did a lot of prayer, theology, and soul searching. We did speeches and papers about ourselves and our spiritual journey. We learned about each other in a very intimate way with no boundaries or false pretenses.

As time went by, folks dropped out of the classroom. I moved from the front of the room to the back because I was the only one at my table. I sat between two guys: Patrick, and Robert. Patrick was a player, and Robert was just fun-

loving and very committed to his wife and family. I just wasn't looking.

One day Chris did a speech on smoking. He had quit because he didn't want that to be something his kids remembered him for. The next week I asked him how it was going. We talked briefly. The following week, he asked me about why women were so insecure? I told him because men give us reasons to be! He told me a little about his ex-wife, that she would check his phone logs, listen to his calls, smell him when he came home, etc. My response was, "What did you do to her to make her so suspicious?"

I told him that I used to be on top of the world; had a great life, great kids, a wonderful home and a decent job. I went on to tell him about how I was blindsided by your father's affair and how I was never able to trust him after that. I told Chris I believed he was responsible for his ex's suspicions.

A few weeks later Patrick dropped out of the class and Chris sat by me. He told me he was approaching his 40th birthday. I was already forty. I told him how significant the age was. In the Bible forty represents all of the major events of the world, suffering that was rewarded, and grace that was earned. I had told him about a book, "The Purpose Driven Life," which was a book a friend of mine gave me for my 40th birthday. From there we just really connected.

I hope this helps you to understand.

Love,
Mom

Now, as I read the words, I would answer with honesty. I was not thinking; I was surviving. I had the grief of also knowing that I allowed dysfunction to grow in my home. I did not provide parameters for stability, although, I wanted to. I wanted the best; I just did not have the formula to allow it to happen.

My granddaughter Savannah was born just six months later and has been the glue that held Erin together over the past few years. She is a blessing. As I watched her birth, I prayed that this generation would have things differently. Like Erin, she has creamy white skin, curly blonde hair, blue eyes and unyielding determination. Erin is raising her in Florida as a single parent, a choice she has made and I am proud. This decision is my hope that life will be better. Erin has the strength to move forward on her own. She has since gone back to school and is slowly pulling the pieces of her life together, yet remains confused about love, mutual respect, and trust.

I accept that some of her anger lies with me. I saw her as a strong child who did not need intervention. I trusted that she would make good decisions on her own. I forgot that every child needs a mother, and my efforts at providing that fell short. One additional thing that I gave her as a mother, something for which the guilt in my heart cannot seem to rest, was a defective heart. When she endured surgery to be fitted for a defibrillator, I was not able to be there for her as I was in the hospital repairing my defective heart as well. I couldn't be there for her, like so many times in her life.

She wanted a mommy, but not this one. She pushed me away as so many kids do. She wanted the mother who allowed her to do whatever she wanted when she was young and a mother who had the health to help with grand parenting. I did not qualify as a parent in her eyes. It is so much easier to look back and see the flaws in what we have done instead of the good. Like Amanda, I may have missed some clues with Erin. Reality is, you can't go back, and you just hope you learn, are forgiven, and then make a valuable connection somewhere else along the way.

Reflection:

My life lessons are no different than anyone else's. We all have our own destiny, our own journey, and we are all intertwined. Just like my heart, I have flaws and do not always function the way others think I should. I wonder, however, if I did would the outcome have been better? While I am walking down my own path, feeling my own pain, learning my own lessons, so is everyone else. I'm not sure at what point in our lives we become responsible for our own decisions and are able to open our eyes to incorporate one another's journeys to become more harmonious in our existence.

My heart was removed from my body because it was not what I needed to survive. It had a diminished function within me, and no function without me. Today, I rely on the heart of someone else to exist. I have not forgotten who I am, where I came from, and the pain I have endured to become who I am today.

I have no survival guilt because I believe God chose me to receive the gift of life and that I still have things to accomplish here. I'm not sure what it is but for now I believe it starts with gestures of kindness and compassion toward one another

The lives of all people flow through time, and regardless of how brutal one moment may be, how filled with grief or pain or fear, time flows through all lives equally.

Orson Steve Cars

A Heart Reborn:

The gift:
I experienced no fear as
My heart began to fail
Embraced by God's
Arms all around me.
Holding
Bringing a loud peace
Carrying me to a Space
Of new birth.
I touch the realism of My soul
The life force that's
Keeping my body ready
To receive the gift…a
NEW Heart donated
To give me a
Second chance at life
As my soul watches
God teaches me to live
Again.

Brenda Butler Hamlett

POTHOLES

Waking up:

I heard my name; I was so peaceful until then. Opening my eyes I saw silhouettes of people around me. "It's Chris, Amanda, Barbara, Cricket, Adam, and Jade," I heard them each recounting their names and I tried to nod acknowledging I was aware of their presence. It was odd to see them all wearing gowns, masks, and gloves and I must've looked puzzled. My lips and throat were dry as I tried to swallow but couldn't because I still had the tube down my throat.

It was hard to comprehend it all but I knew I was alive, no white lights, no beautiful gardens; I was still here with my family and friends! I slept off and on quite a bit and I'm sure I was pretty well-medicated over the next few days. The first day they pulled out my breathing tube and got me out of bed with what reminded me of a baby walker. I was incredibly weak and recall giving Chris a desperate "save me" look. My knees and legs could barely hold me. I was exhausted and tubes were everywhere, but I did it! Later, I was even allowed to try my liquid diet...yum? Chris updated my "blog" as follows:

Day 1 and 2

First, let me apologize to all those people I did not call with the news. As you might imagine, when I received Linda's call things began happening very quickly. When we arrived Wednesday, we were greeted by cameras from ABC News who were there to film the entire "event." Linda went into surgery at about 11:45 p.m. on Wednesday and came out around 5:30 a.m. Thursday. When the surgeon came to the waiting room to talk to us (cameraman in tow), he said that things could not have gone any better. She came out without needing any I.V. medications to keep her blood pressure up, which was a very good sign. He thought that she would be able to be discharged home in a week to ten days.

She remained sedated for the better part of the morning but by the afternoon she was taken off the ventilator, was opening her eyes, and able to talk to everyone. She was getting quite a bit of pain medication to keep her comfortable, which left her very groggy so we left her to rest for the night. Everyone taking care of her was amazed at her progress for the first day.

Today she is much more alert; a great amount of the swelling has gone down and her color looked great. She is going to be getting out of bed today, one her arterial lines will be coming out and the hope is that after she gets up they will be able to remove her chest tubes. She is beginning to receive more to eat and drink, which she is tolerating well. We've been told that we can track her progress by how many things get taken away on a daily basis (I.V. lines, drains, medications, etc.).

As of right now, her progress has been remarkable. I will continue to keep everyone updated, but if I know Linda, she'll be doing her own updates by tomorrow. On another positive note, Dr. Ken went in for his heart yesterday afternoon and is doing well. Our thoughts are with him and his family.

Good Night.
Chris

May 9, 2009

    Hey everyone, it's me! I think Chris did a great job updating so I'll stick to the nuts and bolts. All went incredibly well. I no longer have the central line in my neck, the PICC line in my arm, the arterial line in my arm, or the chest tubes; there were three. I was scared to death when they were pulling those because they made me feel really odd. The doctor moved them around so I could get a feel for what it would be like. I had to take a breath in then "bear down" while they were pulled. I was afraid to pop a suture or something!

    What was really cool is he pulled all three at once so by the time I finished the first breath, all tubes were out. The CVP and arterial line went well too and required the usual pressure to stop bleeding. So I had a few new dressings needless to say. I still had a drain where the defibrillator was and thought it a perk that it is gone! Chris and I joked with the surgeon about resale value of it. It had never fired. I guess the doctor was confused with the humor and started to talk about the "black market" for such things. HMMM?

    Anyway, I had pacing wires that were put in for the new heart, but mine didn't need them. They should come out in a few days. It seemed the new heart and I am going to get along just fine. It's hard to actually feel it beating with all the sutures and dressings, but it was fascinating to hear it beat during the first echo and seeing it move for the first time. If I wasn't in so much pain, I may have cried.

    I liked to look at the EKG monitor now and see my new wave, normal blood pressure and pulse. It was strident and powerful. It made me feel special; especially since I'm not normal.

I giggled trying to type because my "sausage fingers" were not at all dexterous! Someone asked me to cross my fingers yesterday and I couldn't. It's funny to laugh at yourself. As Chris said, the swelling had come down quite nicely and my cheeks have a little color. Some of it is because of the high blood sugars due to all the steroids, but tomorrow will be a better day.

We looked forward to a clean biopsy next week and getting the rest of the tubes out tomorrow. If all goes well, I should be home next weekend. ABC has completed their filming for a few days, so tomorrow should be quieter. For the night, I'll shuffle back into bed and get a good night's sleep.

May 10, 2009

For me it seemed I was spending too much time waiting for things. I wanted a pain pill and waited two hours only to be told I had nothing ordered. I said to the nurse, "C'mon, a fresh post-op?" Gently I asked, "How do you go from Dilaudid injections every three hours to nothing?"

Needless to say, by the time I got something, I was a little agitated. I asked the nurse to close my door so I could settle myself down. At midnight they didn't miss coming in for vitals just a half-hour later. The door once again left open. My room was across from a unit door and the med room, so between codes, call bells, and doors creaking I was losing patience. I rang for the nurse to help me reposition for the night and slept until 4 a.m. vitals.

The nurse came in. "I have your I.V. Lasix, and once I give it, are you ready to have your Foley pulled out (the tube in my bladder)?" she asked.

"You just pumped me with medication to make me pee, and at 4 a.m. gave me pain medicine, and now you want me getting up to go to the bathroom?" I reverberated.

I opted to keep it in until the morning and planned on sleeping with that contraption! Morning came quickly and I had my Foley pulled, my drain pulled, and I.V. pulled. The day started with a chest x-ray, and a bucket of pills. I even had my own med sheets! After my physical therapy assessment, I regained my freedom to walk to the bathroom myself!

By now, the only things left behind were the pacing wires tunneling under my skin and attached to the atria of my heart. They would be used in case they needed to slow down and pace the new heart. I was more alert and focused now and certainly more aware of my new heart's (her) character. I intently listened and focused on its beating as breaths of air filled and exited my chest. She was bold and powerful, yet I'd say a little anxious. I now began the process of wanting to protect her, talking to her, and accepting her. I kept reminding her it's all going to be fine and that we are going to be well-taken care of. I imagined that if an organ had any awareness of where it is, this one would be saying, "Hey, where am I, and who is that voice I keep hearing?"

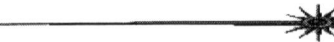

Dr. Ken was doing remarkably well but progressing a little more slowly than I expected, but he was prepared for that. The color in his cheeks appeared rosy and healthy when I peeked in on him. I hoped I could visit again tomorrow if everyone seemed rested.

I walked calmly back to my room feeling blessed yet tired, and needed to rest. I noticed the view was different from this side of the building as I paused to acknowledge it at my bedside. I took the opportunity to rest there briefly preparing for my new acrobatic trick; getting into bed now was like a "stop, drop, and roll," drill! Each effort was getting better.

When I got settled the phone rang. It was Julie calling to congratulate me. She seemed genuinely excited for me yet the call was bittersweet. She was sick at home still waiting.

May 11, 2009

The doctors talked about discharging me on my ninth day out of surgery. I was probably not strong enough for that physically, but psychologically I was ready to leave. My medications were now routine and I began to administer them to myself.

To prepare patients to self-medicate at home, they put us through a training routine first. Staff would bring in a wash basin filled with medication bottles. The patient is expected to match the medications to medication cards. I thought I did great with the first six pills I was taught based on what I read, but there were dose changes since I prepared them.

"These are not correct," the nurse told me.

"Well, as of last evening, I believe they are," I replied. The nurse actually had to check the orders prior to me passing the medication. Thank goodness for electronic medication records to catch our mistakes!

I looked in the mirror to see my cheeks being flushed fairly regularly. I was reminded of Chris' son, thinking he would get a kick out of the fact that one of the meds makes my cheeks flushed, just like his. I told him later on the phone, "You and I are definitely related now. We both have pink cheeks."

At the end of the day I took myself to the lounge where I could watch the sunset. I was visited by Dr. Ken's family. They were holding up remarkably well. He continued to have increased difficulty with his recovery and they seemed exhausted.

It frightened me somewhat that someone I had become so fond of was suffering. I prayed silently for their family and Dr. Ken when they left the room. As I walked, I realized something remarkable: Dr. Ken and I had our surgeries on the same day. What a neat synchronicity!

May 12, 2009

The Physician's assistant came in around 8 a.m. to pull my "pacing lines." Of all that I've experienced, it was probably the most bizarre! My expression must've been priceless as she snipped the sutures and told me I would feel the tugging on my heart as those "dissolvable" sutures let loose. To say the least I was freaked out! It felt if I were being unstitched from the inside out. I understood fully why I was on bed rest afterward.

After four hours, I took a shower for so long that I thought my skin would complain. I ran the water and sat for what seemed like hours. How refreshing not to be attached to a single thing! Of course the flip side was for the first time since the surgery, I saw myself naked. With so many holes and sutures in my body, I resembled a "Raggedy Ann" doll. *Well,* I thought, *gangsters see their scars as badges of courage each telling a story, and I have mine.* Each wound; the result of a well-deserved journey.

I was amazed to learn the chest incision was not sutured or stapled. I was glued! I found humor in the meaning of the expression, "to come unglued!" The incision healed from the inside out and the glue would release though the healing process. I pictured the movie, *Death Becomes Her,* and looked forward to watching my "paint peel." I anticipated being amused by it all.

May 14, 2009

Today, I was in the last mile! Chris, along with my father-in-law Vince arrived to help prepare for my long-awaited return trip home. Like a fine timepiece, Vince counted down the hours. We were scheduled to leave around noon the next day. I was on the schedule for a final biopsy at 10 a.m., but there was an opening at 8 a.m. I was thrilled!

Tiffany, one of the vascular lab nurses, arrived to take me for the procedure. It was great to see her familiar face. When I saw her I knew it was time to go, and hopped happily up onto the gurney with my blanket in hand. She laughed knowing I knew the drill all too well.

The staff there was so excited to see me "on this side of the transplant." I got lots of hugs and well-wishes. Jeff, one of the O.R. techs, let me choose the style of music they played while I was biopsied, and the nurse was amazed that I didn't want to be sedated. I was in and out of there and back to the floor by 8:45 a.m.!

Admittedly, the concept of a biopsy of the heart unnerved me. Access through the jugular was no longer a concern–I was a pro, yet the concept of taking pieces of heart tissue; not so much! It was fascinating to visualize my new heart and its vessels on the monitors. The doctor told me that the results looked promising, the heart was functioning beautifully, and all my values were excellent. The procedure was uneventful, and the results would be ready tomorrow.

Once back, I treated myself to strawberry pancakes for breakfast and went about my busy day. There were so many people involved in discharge planning. I had to see the surgical team, the heart failure team, the transplant team, physical therapy, case management, chaplain services, pharmacy, clinic services, and the news team.

Admittedly, the medication part was a little crazy and a lot to learn. I was up to twenty pills–some supplements, the rest to prevent infection and rejection. I filled my 7-day container for the week, a requirement before leaving, and prepared to go home. WHEW!

In the final preparation, I had another Echo–which was a little painful having that roller press upon my wounds. I thought it was neat to hear the tech say, "It's pretty." He referred to my amazing beating heart. Afterward, I needed a chest x-ray. I waited patiently and at that point had already packed my things and was ready to go.

Chris did the coolest thing. He drove to J.P. Licks, the ice cream store I could see from my window with a wash basin filled with ice and brought back two hot fudge sundaes for Lauren and I! I was so excited to go up there to say goodbye to her and her wonderful family. They gave me a card and a bag of "Snicker's snackers." I may be in a sugar coma from it all but the gesture was priceless.

I said goodbye to everyone possible on the 6th, 9th, and 10th floors including Dr. Ken and his family.

I was relieved knowing he had had his first uneventful day since his surgery. I thought, *My job here is done*. I slept peacefully that night dreaming about returning home.

May 15, 2009

"Good morning, we are finally going home!" Chris said as he leaned forward to kiss me on the cheek. We were entwined into each other's eyes, gazing lovingly. A few moments later the morning routine began. Everything was right on schedule. I had my final EKG, pharmacy teaching, and flurry of discharge planners. There were lots of smiles and hugs all around. I spoke with my friend Kenny who was so kind to call to say goodbye.

The nurse Debbie came in with my biopsy results.

Drum roll please...the biopsy results showed massive rejection!

"Linda, you are rejecting the new heart so significantly it warrants you staying in the hospital a little longer," Debbie delivered the news.

I don't think I, Chris, or his Dad could've been any more shocked! I have to admit, I understand that this is part of the process, but I was truly blind sighted, I felt great until then. It was then I thought I would buckle at the knees and fall apart.

I held it together long enough to hear the plan for three days of I.V. steroids and a repeat biopsy the next Thursday.

I did allow the newsman to tape this part of the interaction because this is a very real part of this process, and if I am part of the documentary, felt people would need to know this happens. I wanted people to know that transplantation it is a lifelong process that doesn't end with surgery. In fact several people had told me, "You exchange one bucket of problems for another."

Once the news team left I had to send Chris and his father home because I knew he had to get back to the boys. We hadn't planned for this. I went into self-protect mode until I could better grasp what was going on: until I could face that I was following the path of my sister Patti. My head spun in a whirlwind. I needed him to leave so I could fall apart alone.

It was the single most difficult thing I ever had to do; lying that I was fine with him leaving me behind. I wanted to sob in his arms, be held and nurtured, yet I had always put myself second. He didn't want to go but I knew he had no choice. When our eyes locked it was clear we were both in agony.

I shed a lot of tears of disappointment with him and fell apart like a shattered abandoned child when he left. I knew

I had to work through it, but had fallen to an all- time low. I had allowed myself to care so much about my new family, my life, and getting back to the ones I love that I was devastated when I couldn't. I was angry at myself for caring so much; for setting myself up for that level of pain.

I was fortunate that several support persons stopped by to see me allowing me to release my pain, express my sadness, and just cry. They just allowed me to feel the pain and it was O.K.

When I was able to regroup the next day I realized that I was fortunate for many things. In this case, I was young, fairly healthy, and I had a great immune system which is what most people need. Just like the rest of my life, it needed to be kicked down a little so that we, me, and my new heart, can get along. I am fortunate I found out while I was still there allowing rejection to get nipped in the bud. I was certainly glad I didn't have to make an extra trip back to the hospital. That thought was untathomable!

The heart itself is well and had no damage which is a blessing. I committed to spending some time being kind to myself, reflecting on my faith, and remembering how far I had come in such a short period of time. There was another beautiful sunset and tomorrow was another day.

Reflection:

I believe that the more difficult and painful a life experience, the greater our potential for personal and spiritual growth. Although many of the crises I have endured appear excruciating and full of disappointment, I freely accept them. I am often amazed at the strength I have gained and the ability I have developed to support others in difficult situations. It is in this I have discovered my greatest achievements, and I know I am where God wants me to be.

The greatest Christians in history seem to say that their sufferings ended up bringing them closest to God–so this is the best thing that could happen, not the worst.

Perry Kreeft

Chapter 12

A Fight to the End

The immune system not only fights infections, it also defends the body against foreign objects that should not be there, like a transplanted organ. This sophisticated system reacts to offending germs by creating antibodies to attack them. If allowed, the immune system could destroy an organ, a process called rejection.

To prevent this from occurring with a transplanted organ, medications are utilized to minimize the threat of the immune system to that organ. There is a fine balance between suppressing the immune response to prevent rejection and allowing for the body to become too weakened to fight other infections such as the common cold or viruses. In fact, there are viruses that we have previously been exposed to which lie dormant in our bodies and may recur when the immune system is compromised.

In life when a threat to what we know is safe occurs our reaction, just like the immune system, is to strike out against the danger, for if we ignored it, it could be allowed to fester to the point of destruction.

The unattended "organisms" in my marriage brought about painful, infectious wounds. There was no fight to preserve my family, just acceptance of the intruder's presence: left untreated. Over time, just as the body deteriorates and the heart weakens, so did my marriage. The *stability I thought I had attained with my children had become quicksand.*

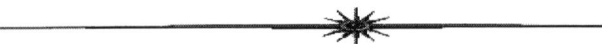

Adam was my pride and joy, my boy and what I knew would be the last child in our perfect family. In reality he was the child who pointed out my responsibility for my marriage dissolving. I had spent years blaming Ray for having affairs, but Adam helped me to see the truth. I never invited Ray into our marriage, and was not able to.

As an infant, Adam was content requiring only the simplest of his needs met to be happy. Perhaps knowing he had two sisters was all it took; maybe he sensed my exhaustion and drained energy having three small children.

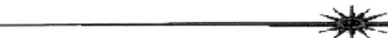

On Amanda's 4th birthday, when I was trying to get the house and kids ready for company, I realized how much I had nurtured Ray's maladaptive parenting. I had been up most of the night baking and cleaning, and was exhausted. When morning came, I made our traditional weekend family breakfast which we all looked forward to. To me it was the one thing that brought us together as a family. Once everyone was finished, I sent the girls to get ready while I attempted to clean up. I placed Adam (we nicknamed him "Addy") in the baby swing and Ray went to lie down on the couch watching television.

Looking around at all the dishes, I was a little distraught. The clock was ticking. Our guests would arrive shortly. I had placed a great deal of pressure on myself to make the day perfect. Not only was it Amanda's birthday, but it would be the first time that many of our friends and family would see our new baby. Adam was only six weeks old.

Erin came into the kitchen tugging on my jeans. "Uppy (up) mommy?" she asked wanting to be held.

Amanda followed behind Erin with her birthday dress on crooked and her hand caught in the sleeve, and then Adam began to cry. I began to feel a little out of control and needed Ray's help. I was afraid of appearing weak and unable to handle the situation with my babies that I so desperately enjoyed. I took a deep breath, set Erin down for a moment and picked up Adam and handed him to Ray.

At that moment, I saw how awkward, almost uncomfortable he was holding our baby. I realized that I had not involved him in caring for any of his children, not simply because he hadn't been there, but because I hadn't allowed it. Instead, I tolerated him joining his buddies at the bar after his ten-hour workdays and enabled him to miss all of the family rituals. He missed our dinners together, he missed playtime, bath time, story time, and bedtime kisses. I felt awful that Ray had been neglected in the everyday joyful experiences that draw couples together. I did not learn to trust or rely on another person in my life and he didn't learn to be a father. We were not a family, just people living in the same house independently growing apart.

I wished I could recapture the time and admit my vulnerability. Perhaps if I had, we could've fallen in love all over again while relying on one another's strengths and accepting our weaknesses. Life may not have been harmonious, but we would have managed. We could have grown old together. Instead we never tried.

Adam grew as a typical boy as far as playing sports, playing with cars, playing with snakes and frogs. Adam always wanted to share his slimy friends with me and brought them in the house proudly.

"Here mommy," he said one day showing me a snake he caught in the yard.

Thank goodness Ray was there to get it from him and return it outside.

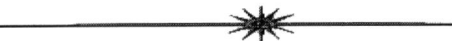

When he was old enough he played baseball and football in the town leagues. Initially it was me teaching him to throw a ball and the basic fundamentals of sports, but as he got older he needed his father for the skills.

It was then I noticed Ray was able to give more of himself and becoming more actively involved as a parent. It seemed he appreciated feeling needed and I once again mourned for the past. There were so many "ifs" in our lives: if life simply could have been different, if I had allowed Ray to be a parent then at his young age of nineteen.

Adam grew to love sports and excelled in them, which made us proud as parents. He developed a unique personality and wonderful friendships that lasted through his adulthood. It was rare that Adam would be home. In his free time he was out somewhere in the neighborhood with friends. There was always a planned event in our neighborhood.

He and his friend Ryan spent years building a fort in the backyard. Their carpentry skills improved as they grew older and I wondered if he was trying to build a house where he could store his dreams of stability.

By the time he was eighteen-years-old, the fort had turned into a two-story with windows and a balcony. He and his friends began making home-made movies up in the fort, starting with classics such as Romeo and Juliet. Later, their films expanded into neighborhood action films. We would watch hysterically laughing at some of the stunts, embarrassed by him riding a bicycle through a local store in a "Speedo," and fearful when he jumped from roofs and trees. I loved his confident and fun-loving disposition as well as his creativity and ability to occupy himself.

He went through a rough spell around the age of ten when he spent an entire summer sick or broken somehow. We started with scarlet fever, then seven sutures in his foot from dropping a metal glider on it. A few weeks later he went to his friend Steve's.

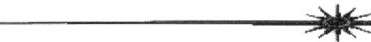

It was a beautiful summer day and I dropped him off. I loved that he was so self-reliant and had so many friends whose parents enjoyed having him over. As I pulled my white Buick into the driveway back home, the house phone rang. I hurriedly went in to answer it. It was Steve's little sister, Lindsey. She was around five-years-old.

"Ms. Bo pee," she said struggling to pronounce the name, "Adam got cut on a tree and mom wants you to come here."

"I'll be there as soon as I can, don't worry honey," I said.

I hung up the phone and got back in my car. When I turned down the street to Steve's house, I saw ambulances near the neighbor's house and I hoped everything was alright, never realizing the ambulance was there for Adam.

When I got to the backyard I saw Adam impaled to a tree. He was alert and holding back tears in front of his friend. They had been making stairs for Steve's treehouse when he fell, landing on a nail that had punctured his abdomen. The paramedics, unsure if there was any internal damage, pried him away from the tree with a crowbar, 2x4 board and all. Once the board was secured with gauze around his entire torso, we rode off in the ambulance.

Adam was always a brave little man and comforted me more than anything. He was a "hit" in the E.R. The doctors x-rayed him with the board intact; it was an x-ray to remember. It showed the board and multiple nails that had been hammered into it, many bent as you would expect from "child carpenters."

"Well, the nail Adam impaled himself with is one that actually caught under the bone of his ribcage; it must've been supporting his weight. He was very lucky." I was so relieved and thanked him and God for good news. Today, Adam refers to the puncture scar as a bullet wound, which I guess sounds more impressive. I still have the x-ray.

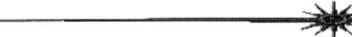

Adam has grown into a respectful young man with character and integrity. When I left his father, it was the hardest thing I ever did. I wished Adam had come with me, but deep down, I knew that an 18-year-old boy needs his father. He could've let the experience infect our lives, fester and grow, but instead Adam simply asked for an explanation. I am grateful for that and it is something I can only now give. I told him I was broken and needed to find myself. I had made mistakes, poor choices, and bad decisions and needed to pull myself together in order to be a better person. I was living a lie appearing happy for the sake of raising them in a two-parent household. I no longer wanted them to learn from my dysfunction. I wanted them to know it was not anyone's fault and that his Dad and I had made our decisions when we were very young, and our lives had been spent developing patterns that I didn't want repeated in his life. I tried further to explain that I was not able to see clearly, and living there imprisoned me.

Maybe if I had learned this sooner, I would have recognized that the fort being built on the outside needed to be built first in the hearts of people inside. I only began to scratch the surface of understanding then.

The truth I can see now is the truth of the divine, "Love one another as I have loved you." When we live for the good of others, and do not accept negative patterns in our lives, we begin to grow. Looking back, if Ray and I had only nurtured one another as well as our children, we would today be watching our grandchildren climb in the fort that their "Uncle Addy" built. They would be building simple dreams cherished over a lifetime.

I look back at my children now, at ages older than when Ray and I met. I hope they can learn from our mistakes, forgive, and move on. The truth is now and will always be, that they are loved by the two people who created them.

I am grateful that Adam asked the questions he did and I am thrilled to have the relationship with him that I have today. My fear of rejection had instead been replaced by his strength, acceptance, and support. I pray for his continuing support as I am still learning...searching for my path.

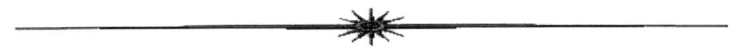

Reflection:

As we grow personally and spiritually, we are thankful for those opportunities in which we are allowed to express ourselves as an individual, to be listened to, and to be understood whether or not others agree with our actions. I had that opportunity and I am eternally grateful.

As a parent, we tend to give everything we have and expect little in return. Reversing this understanding, however, our children are not always intellectually capable of processing the complexities of adult decisions as we often expect them to. Yet, they can surprise us when they are called upon. My children were no exception.

In my case, they initially rebelled when my marriage to their dad fell apart, rejecting me—equally devastating as my heart rejection. Yet with proper treatment, both were able to manage. I am thankful that I waited to end my relationship with Ray until my children were older and more able to share their feelings with me. Yes, it was incredibly painful for all of us, but there was never a moment I didn't know exactly where I stood with each of them. Our love for our children will always be as strong as the beat of a healthy heart.

Our real blessings often appear to us in the shape of pains, losses, and disappointments; but let us have patience and we soon shall see them in their proper figures.

Joseph Addison

The Heart Fallen Victim to Rejection:

The body's defense systems are incredibly efficient as it is able to immediately react to offending invaders. It will attack with a vengeance; its intent to destroy. When this response is directed specifically at a transplanted organ, it is called rejection. If the defense system's attack is not halted in a timely manner, the result could be certain damage and eventual death to that organ. Our innate abilities to protect and defend the body are not designed to recognize that the organ it is indeed attacking is crucial to its survival.

The organ recipient may not recognize there is any problem in the initial phases of rejection when the white blood cells are destroying tissue, other than perhaps feeling tired or having cold symptoms and it may not be until much later before professional help is sought.

Organ rejection, similar to emotional rejection, can be devastating to the overall well-being of its victim. In both cases, while the inability to recognize rejection is occurring, allowing it to continue long-term can result in the demise of the individual; the cessation of life.

May 16, 2009

I am having a much better day emotionally. My steroids are making me a little puffy and my skin began to feel a little tight. I felt like a sausage packed into its casing. I convinced myself the drugs should be bottled for cosmetic injection because they have "puffed" the wrinkles out from around my eyes. I actually looked years younger–radiant and exuberant.

My mood, to me, seemed a little edgy, in fact like a tyrant, but Chris told me otherwise. Secretly, I acknowledged that he loved me enough to spare my feelings and was smart enough to know better than to say anything else. In order to cope, I had found that the intensity of the medication could be reduced with vigorous physical activity.

The "Pike," was a corridor interconnecting the buildings of the hospital that stretched along Francis Street. I began to refer to it as, "the mile," remembering the movie, *The Green Mile,* with Tom Hanks. I would endearingly recant to Chris, "Walking the mile, walking the mile," as we recalled seeing the prisoners do in the movie. I tried my hardest to plan ahead by exhausting myself walking before each dose of I.V. steroids. I felt like a caged animal ready to attack with great impulsivity, and feeling out of control. The medications caused such an intense mania that I felt I was on high alert. On them, it was difficult to rest; my mind raced, and my muscles couldn't rest. I reminded myself that this was indeed what I needed to do in order to survive. For me, it was a psychological escape, knowing in the end, it would be worth it!

Dr. Givertz stopped in with some great news. My heart was doing well, the echo showed no damage and the function remained excellent. I had even noticed that despite the "jitters" from the steroids, the heart–my new heart, felt calmer. I again envisioned the heart's awareness of its surroundings. "Why are you hurting me?" It would ask me.

I talked to it, telling it all will be fine, yet it wasn't the case. My body was having a "brute force attack" against it.

Though rejection is out of my control, I feel somehow guilty, as though somehow I'd failed to protect it; just like my inner child and my daughter. I scorned my immune system for attacking our only hope for survival. Mentally I asked it, *How can you not recognize that this is what we have waited so long for?* My body was being an impolite host to our guest, and because the guest was going to stay permanently, we needed to treat it like family.

I was thankful for medications to help me, and understood that the best contribution I could make was to take the medicine and take care of my body. Yes, I was afraid of the horrific side effects, but recognized I had come too far to give in; too far to repeat patterns from so long ago. If it is God's will and I surrendered to it, I had complete faith that the rest would follow.

The tremors themselves made my body feel as though it was on "vibration" mode. I was experiencing an internal restlessness and inability to sit still or remain calm. I coped by convincing myself the vibration was like a baby being rocked in a cradle, visualized myself as an infant, and allowed myself to be lulled into a beautiful slumber.

Some evenings were more difficult than others to settle myself and I found myself relying on my relaxation techniques: meditation or melodic, relaxing music. I found a television channel called, the "Care Station," which I truly enjoyed. It had wonderful scenes from nature both on earth and in the skies. Utilizing all of my resources, I would find I was in a calmer place before the medication thus more readily able to capture some much needed rest afterward.

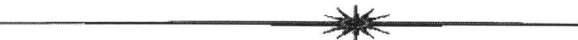

After I woke, called to tell me Julie was once again in the hospital and asked if I could stop by her room to see her. When I did I was exuberant about it being her turn soon and an end in sight for her too.

"Look!" I said, "just a few days out and I feel amazing." I rambled on and on yet Julie sat quietly.

"Linda, I won't be getting a heart," she paused, "they took me off the list because they won't be able to find a match." She told me holding back tears.

"What does that mean? What will they do for you?" I was puzzled.

"They will send me home to die," she confirmed.

I tried to process what she had to say, tried to come up with some words of wisdom, yet I wasn't prepared. I started to cry with her.

"I am so sorry, is there anything I can do?" I hugged her for a period of time and told her I would continue to contact her. "Don't hesitate if you need anything…anything," I reinforced.

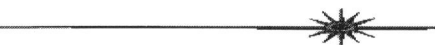

The walk back to my room was slow and quiet. I was so fortunate for my chance at life. I prayed for Julie and her family hoping for peace, and then fell asleep.

I often woke up early in the morning to the brilliance of the rising sun. It made me feel grateful and refreshed. I would complete some morning rituals, which included engulfing my "bucket of meds," (a term I got from Kenny). Despite all of the activities I found to occupy myself, sometimes it just seemed there was too much time alone.

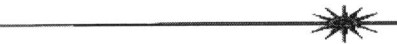

    I reflected on the day I got the original biopsy results, the car was packed with all of my belongings and Chris and his father headed back to New York with all of my belongings. At the time, I was so distraught that mentally I wanted everyone to leave so I could fall apart alone. I was in no mental state to realize I had no clothes, no toiletries, and comforts from home. I thought briefly about buying myself a pair of pajamas or something to make me feel "normal." I envisioned myself as my own version of *Little Orphan Annie*, a role I was comforted in.
Even after all I had been through, I still struggled with asking for help and appearing weak. Although I was self-preserving, once again I shut the ones I loved out. I knew I needed to work on that, and found that in my darkest times, I learned the most and had profound spiritual growth.

    The depth of my thoughts was interrupted by a welcomed visit from Surrinder. She brought with her a beautiful card and friendship mug that she had purchased in the gift shop for me. I was so touched by the sentiment and grateful for my "angel in disguise." I asked her to join me in the little "hospitality area" I had created within my room. I had set up two chairs with a small table between them. On the table, I placed a basket with tea, cocoa, and basic snacks I had collected so I could feel at home with my visitors. Our conversation over tea was one that will leave a lasting impression.

We spoke about Dr. Ken and I was elated to hear he had been moved out of the unit to the 7th floor. They had been through so much together, and the relief on her face was unmistakable. As Surrinder spoke, I thought about how much I admired her (and her family), as they remained diligently supportive of one another at Dr. Ken's bedside. It was truly beautiful.

Later, Geoff and Sheila popped in. I was awestruck to see how well they were doing. He announced they had set a date to get married in August 2009, and it was a thrill to see the energy radiating from them as they spoke. I envisioned him doing the "Funkie Chicken" dance, as he spoke of the traditions they had planned for their wedding. I had forgotten how much I enjoyed his sense of humor! After all of the recent struggles, emotion, loss, and love, here they were planning a grand occasion.

Kenny also called to check in on me all the way from his summer home in Maine! I was elated to hear from him and loved listening to the stories of his days on the beach. I reflected that soon enough, it would be me. Kenny sometimes referred to his wife Nancy, as his "sidekick," which makes me laugh. I loved how much of an interest he and his family had taken to sharing in my life. When I hung up the phone I realized, all of the transplant patients suffered joys and disappointments as one.

My sister Joyce called then to share stories about her wedding, which took place the day before. She intrigued me with all of her crazy little "quirky" dilemmas. She said the wedding was beautiful with the exception of my nephew speaking up at the moment the Pastor asked, "If there is anyone who believes this couple should not be joined."

"Stop! You're ruining your lives!" Perry screamed running in circles.

I burst out laughing, not really sensitive to my sister's chagrin at the time. And regardless, the wedding continued.

Sometimes I was angry that life marched on with or without me and very secretly I wished just maybe I was important enough that they could wait for me to be there. It was selfish, but I wanted to be there to celebrate along with those I loved. Still, I was very happy that she found love and was able to restart her life.

The chaplain, Katherine, made an especially welcomed trip to my room at the end of the day. We shared some inspirational moments and prayers which eased my mind just a little. I recognized that I am in a really good place and thankful for each moment that God has granted that I am alive. I have been blessed with sunny days and rainbows, peace with God, and harmony within.

May 17, 2009

It was a little dreary in Boston due to rain most of the day. It didn't stop me from popping my head outside the building for a few minutes though. I actually appreciated the smell of the rain in the city and observed the blossoms on the trees. I walked the "Pike" a few times that day to work off a little "steroid energy." I had the cutest little cherub face and pot-belly started from the meds, but I knew it would be temporary. I warned Chris to let the family, especially the boys, know I would look different when I returned home.

I recalled the first time I'd seen my sister Patti after her transplant. I struggled with the fact that her appearance was so distorted and unfamiliar to me (similar to my Mom's when she had her teeth extracted). In fact, it was difficult for me to look at her and see the sister I once knew and loved. That was until she spoke.

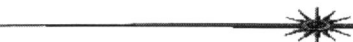

I went to the gift shop briefly to browse and decided to treat myself to a t-shirt to wear with my hospital pants. Without my clothes, once again I found that I became a creative genius! I found a few different prints in the Brigham fabric and began designing outfits. With the help of a little hospital tape, I was able to create cropped pants and peasant-like tops. I struggled with the fact that it was so time-consuming to create clothes that were one-time wear.

I was ecstatic with the kindness and generosity of Lauren's family when Jackie, Lauren's mom stopped by with a bag of freshly laundered, matched outfits, socks, underwear, and even a pair of flip-flops!

"Here you go; we can't have you up here with no clothes; Lauren just won't allow it," she said. "I matched a few outfits I thought you might like and purchased some socks and panties. Let me know if there is anything else you need and when you need me to launder them for you," she continued

"Thank you," I said teary-eyed.

"It is the least we could do for you. Sleep well," she finished, and left.

After she left, I brought the scent of the laundry to my face to take it all in; I loved that familiar home-like smell. I began to cry. I hadn't been mothered in many, many years and desperately missed that.

I began to try on all the outfits as if I had gone shopping and planned what I would wear each day.

I said a prayer for Lauren and her family that their wait would soon be over. I looked forward to her being well on her way to recovery and on with her life. She had such a beautiful presence and a gentle soul.

Later, I walked again, only to find an amazing looking Dr. Ken, waving me into his room. I respected him immensely and often worried about him. My greatest fear came when they could not get him stabilized and had to cardiovert his new heart. Today though, was different. The medical team concluded that the ultimate resolution for Dr. Ken was to implant a pacemaker. Today, and for the first time since we met, I looked upon a man with pink cheeks, a healthy posture, and a confident smile. Such a beautiful smile! His spirit soared and so too did his family! How wonderful it felt to see their joy.

I headed back to my room remembering tomorrow was the day the medical team would meet with me to discuss my plan. I was saddened, Chris was at home with the boys now, but excited to know that my son Adam and his friend Jade were on their way to visit. It was another great day to be alive and for that moment, the tremors and mood swings seemed insignificant.

As I continued to walk, I heard mumblings that yet another transplant was performed. HIPAA prevented anyone from confirming it, so I walked into that unit to see if a name was posted and it was! To my chagrin it wasn't Lauren, yet I knew the name. It was Phil a fairly new patient I had met just a few days before my transplant. He was twenty-eight and his illness sudden. I empathized with his frustration yet secretly felt blessed that I had so much more time to prepare. I prayed that all went well for him and his family, yet yearned for it to be Lauren's turn.

May 18, 2009

Today was my two-week post-op anniversary! I looked at myself amazed at how far I had come and how good I looked despite the rejection. I started the day leisurely because I was NPO for my biopsy. I slept until 3:30 a.m. but was amazed that I fell back to sleep until almost 7 a.m.! Despite all the continued tremors, which worsened when I completed any focused activities like eating or even typing, I found it humorous. It was a small thing in the grand scheme of it all.

I associated it much like having Parkinson's disease or its symptoms and utilized the knowledge to better empathize with the patients I have cared for. Otherwise I felt great, and I took it and ran with it!

My medication levels were checked at 8 a.m. so there was no sense getting up and into the shower until after. I would do my usual walk, but took it easier because the

POTHOLES

cardiac catheter lab for my biopsy was backed up. I was told the machinery was down so I knew there would be delays; usually long ones. Without being able to eat, I opted not to walk to prevent feeling dizzy or lightheaded. I didn't want to fall on my head!

The doctors came in with discouraging news after they reviewed my records in team report. "All four samples of heart tissue biopsy last week significant for severe rejection; the worst we have seen. After re-evaluating your case, we have decided the best course of action was a more aggressive anti-rejection option. It involves more I.V. medication and a longer stay," I was told

With a disheartened sigh, I continued to listen.

"The medication is called OKT3 which had significant risks and side effects, but we feel it is the best course of action," Dr. Desai told me.

I was unable to process anything he said after that. I had frozen emotionally in much the same way I did twenty years ago.

This was the medication I knew too well. The infamous day my sister Patti was emergency flown home from North Carolina. I recalled vividly, Michelle her case manager's words from so long ago, "OKT3, cardiac arrest, resuscitate...another heart." It was all a blur. I never forgot the dead silence at the other end of the phone, never forgot the name of the medication, and never forgot not saying goodbye to my sister. To this day, I regret not insisting Ray watch the kids so that I could have been there with her.

Fast forward twenty years, and here I was making that same decision, and this time I was alone. History was repeating itself, there were no other options, and quite frankly I too could die. I felt it was senseless to worry, and that I had come way too far to die. I agreed to the treatment never telling Chris what I knew.

I was sent for an MRI prior to the medication to assess the damage from my rejection. It took about an hour. I was admittedly surprised that it was nothing like I had anticipated. Claustrophobia wasn't a concern, and I didn't require sedation, but it was noisy! Even with the music and the headphones on the noise wasn't banging like people described, it was like being in a pinball machine! The camera reminded me of a foghorn when it took pictures, often startling me. I had to hold my breath on and off for long periods of time; it was a workout–especially with fresh incisions in my chest and being so out of shape!

During portions of the MRI I cried, and for the rest I fought back tears. My emotions overwhelmed me and I felt safe in that tunnel crying where no one could see. I could blame it on the music, songs like Fleetwood Mac's, "Landslide," but it wasn't the case.

Dr. Ken had a few complications that day and was quite fatigued. We were both in the vascular lab at the same time for different procedures. I went in for my biopsy. As I was being wheeled down the hall I heard my name as he called to me. He was right behind me being transported for his procedure. I gave him big thumbs up and all the nurses laughed.

"Do you two have to do everything at the same time?" they said remembering we had our transplants on the same day. I did pray that God give him some of my positive energy to help him through.

My biopsy went well and I was sedated despite not asking for it. I admit I enjoyed the induced ability to relax. When I returned to my room I could not wait to eat! My weight was down 3.8 pounds from what I felt was starvation but I felt great! Once rested, I made the rounds to visit all of my friends that evening, perhaps for comfort or afraid if anything happened I would not get to say goodbye. Too often people had left my life far too quickly.

Afterward, I walked quietly to the lounge to reflect and watch a sunset. I knew I had an uphill climb ahead of me and just needed to connect with God. I surrendered to Him, knowing He had a bigger plan, hoping to keep my expectations in check. I desperately want to go home but know I need to be healthy enough to do that.

Although I felt today had been a rainbow of emotions, it didn't compare to what I felt Lauren must've been experiencing. Her entire peer group had been transplanted and she remained. She was now approaching 100 days in the hospital and I prayed that God would find the "perfect heart for her" soon. After I completed that thought I recognized that maybe God's plan was that I was still there for her surgery which would make my journey among my transplant family complete.

The biggest obstacle I have struggled with my entire journey is feeling safe and protected. The care here is phenomenal and there is great concern for my well-being. It is a great place to be but I still struggle inside.

I reflected the words of inspiration from my loved ones, remembering the foundation of my support system: my faith, family, and friends. I asked "Disappointment and Frustration" to leave my room. I needed to wipe it from my slate visually in order to move forward. In its place I needed to believe and trust.

May 19, 2009

The doctors came in bright and early giving me the results of the MRI. My cardiac pressures and function remained great and the heart continued to function well without damage. They were pleased I physically appeared well with no clinical symptoms–a great sign. The MRI however showed significant swelling in the heart. I was told this was typical and should resolve as the rejection comes under control and the aggressive plan was to begin.

The next dose of I.V. steroid was followed with a large dose of Benadryl and Tylenol to prevent side effects from the new therapy. The activity heightened around me in spite of my sleepiness from the medication. You also know it's serious by the number of ancillary services that come through the door.

The doctors worried about anaphylactic shock (an allergic reaction), high fevers, pulmonary hypertension, and flu-like symptoms; I was afraid to die but found comfort knowing the first injection was done by a physician at the bedside along with constant monitoring. I had a whole team of doctors standing at my bedside with a protocol in hand. I knew it was my only option.

Of course the nurse had to start another I.V. line in front of all of the doctors. I could tell she was under duress. The poor thing! I had to admit she was very smart because she didn't mess with the little veins and went for the large, juicy ones!

While at the bedside, I heard them talking confirming the medications needed. Right then, it all became incredibly real; I wanted Chris! I hadn't been honest with him and by my choice I was now afraid of dying alone.

The moment had arrived. Now, with I.V. diuretics, an Epi-pen, crisis meds, suction, and oxygen we were all ready. This was the point I closed my eyes and again placed myself in the palm of God's hands.

The medication was intended to wipe out my T-cells and my entire immune system. It is meant to rid me of all of my antibodies, which meant that I would have to be isolated in my room to avoid germs. To prepare, I borrowed some movies and grabbed some books from the library. I had done it before and was ailing to do it again. I went back to my "jail analogy" to self-preserve telling myself for this week my parole had been denied!

Reflection:

Rejection had been the theme of my childhood foundation, innate as the heart's ability to pump and the immune system's ability to fight infection. I became my own immune system willing to protect and attack at all costs. Like white blood cells, I encased myself in my protective covering to prevent myself from being wounded. With this coping mechanism, I prevented myself from being able to love or trust. Although it worked to get me to this point in my life, it was at this most difficult time that I sacrificed what I needed–the security of Chris's warm hand. I neglected to allow my husband to make an informed decision about being with me at a time of chaos. Once again, I endured alone reverting to my comfort zone of so long ago. Despite all of Chris's love and sacrifices to this point, I was afraid; perhaps to let go, perhaps of disappointment. I wish I had taken the chance.

Adversity is not simply a tool. It is God's most effective tool for the advancement of our spiritual lives. The circumstances and events that we see as setbacks are oftentimes the very things that launch us into periods of intense spiritual growth. Once we begin to understand this, and accept it as a spiritual fact of life, adversity becomes easier to bear.

Charles Stanley

POTHOLES

Chapter 13

Beating to a Different Beat

A heart that is beating abnormally may be corrected by medication, pacing, cardio version or even defibrillation. Medication can be used to alter the chemical exchanges in the body to help the heart work better or even contract stronger.

A pacemaker may be implanted to intervene when the heart fails to pump normally, misses a beat, or a beat is weakened or imperceptible. The beauty of a pacemaker is that parameters are programmed in it so that it functions in situations that are identified to create the best possible outcome in situations that may be dangerous. Cardio version is used when a prolonged abnormal heart rhythm needs to be converted back to normal.

In our modern world, another device called a defibrillator can save a life in the event the heart falls into a life-threatening arrhythmia. Defibrillators can have multiple functions including pacemaking, defibrillation, and cardio version.

My previous married life seemed to have many failed attempts at preservation despite valiant effort. Furthermore, my heart was failing and would require surgical intervention. I would survive, my first marriage would not.

POTHOLES

From the beginning, Ray and I had everything and nothing at all. We had everything because we had each other, but we had nothing because we did not know it. We were kids trying to grow up together with three kids in tow. I did not have the wisdom to know that asking him to be responsible, would build responsibility. I never asked him to change his ways when he went out with the boys. I thought he would see that I was not a nagging wife so he would love me more. Instead, he felt unloved and not needed. We had made many mistakes together, the worst being Ray's infidelity and my acceptance of it.

Ray and I tried to make a go of a bad situation though we did not have a solid foundation for marriage. Eventually, Ray left his girlfriend and I felt victorious. If our relationship was based on true faith and love, I would have realized that my thought process was broken. I was not victorious, I was cheated. We could have spoken about remorse, but the words never came. Instead, we did not speak at all. Words were not spoken for we knew the truth. Ray was staying with me because it was too expensive to get divorced and he liked his patterns. A divorce would take effort. The cost of a divorce, displacement of living quarters, and paying child support was too much for Ray. He would rather be stuck with me and I was thrilled. I still clung to the house we lived in and believed we could create a home.

I decided the marriage would be worth the effort if we both tried. I wanted to seek counseling so we could learn to communicate, but Ray didn't believe in it. I was able to forgive what had happened, but feelings of mistrust were imbedded in my broken heart. I never forgot. Every time he was late from work, was out a little too long, or couldn't account for his whereabouts, I wondered, and then regressed to my childhood insecurities. Slowly, I was going insane!

I did take some responsibility for the fact that he said he was lonely when I worked nights. I took responsibility for the fact that between working and kids I had little left to offer. Maybe my role, allowing him to come and go as he pleased, caused him to feel as though I didn't care. Maybe he saw it as a green light. Maybe I had created this monster!

I made more money than Ray; this offended him. He felt guilty and he made several comments about me changing the environment. I did not want us to grow apart, so I changed jobs. When you love someone as much as I loved him, you will sacrifice whatever you can. I took a position that made less money, a day shift, so I could be a wife again to him; the change I made for us didn't matter in the end.

One day, I drew enough courage to mention my feelings to a coworker who told me that I was not responsible for his actions and that I needed to free myself.

She said, "We all answer to God for what we do." After giving her advice a great deal of thought in 1996, I decided to try new things. I found comfort in meeting new friends and creating my own experiences, experiences that felt good and seemed to fill a void in my life. I thought maybe I wanted to be more like Ray and have fun too!

A group of people I worked with went out regularly. Our kids were older now so I decided to join my new friends for happy hour. Somehow I wanted to believe Ray should not be the only one having fun. Happy hour led to wanting more but not bars or booze–just more learning to love life without him. The bar scene was not the example I wanted to set for our children and I was smart enough to know that.

I did learn to ski and was quite proud of how skillfully I mastered it. I loved the cool air in my face, the crisp night air and the sound of my thoughts "swish-swishing" in my head to the rhythm of the skis. I found it to be incredibly cleansing and loved the thrill of learning the hills, the jumps, and the moguls. I loved the physical challenge and the feeling of accomplishment just working up a great sweat. I went on Friday nights religiously to the ski slopes and whenever else I had time for this new joy. I delighted in the different challenges offered on the slopes in Ellicottville and used my season passes whenever time allowed. There was a thrill at reaching the bottom of a hill when the conditions were icy and sheer pleasure in the spring when the warmth of the sun allowed you to ski in shorts!

There were times when I asked Ray and my kids to join us. Ray did agree on one occasion and it did not go well. Overall, he seemed to dislike the sport in general; especially accepting direction from me. We bickered on and off that night and he never went with me again, and I didn't offer to have him join me in a sport I hoped we could've been passionate about. I was learning to love life without him.

I learned to snowmobile a few years later and was thrilled to purchase my own sled. My first sled was a flawless Artic Cat Jag. It was sleek-black with a tinted windshield and bright-colored decals. I rode mainly with a group of guys, so I learned to "ride like the big boys," and with that came learning to detail the sled and engine, change my own spark plugs, and even load/unload it on the trailer myself. I became very self-reliant, and I was proud of myself. I actually felt good in my snowmobile gear.

When we were out sledding, the helmet shielded me from the world. With the hum of the motor underneath me I could be alone with my thoughts. I could sing my heart out, talk to myself and God, or just enjoy being a part of the group. Once again I asked Ray to join but he had no interest in riding the trails.

I tried to explain my enthusiasm saying, "Out there it was a whole new world with its own street signs and possibilities." But it didn't interest him.

Ray decided to buy his own sled but not to be with me. He would not ride the trails with my friends and I.

He would on occasion agree to spend time with me riding together around our home and in the fields nearby. This was the extent of his participation with me. Winter became one of my favorite times of year in Buffalo and I had fallen back into my old routine of having a "date" every weekend by proxy. Not with someone I loved, by people in general.

There were nights we went out to local bars for the evening specials. There were clam nights, wing nights, and even karaoke. I loved to sing and dance so I participated with everything I had. I didn't care what anyone thought, my kids were growing to be very independent, Amanda was now in high school and Erin and Adam were in middle school. They were involved in their friends and activities, often in bed while I was recapturing my life.

I joined a gym and worked out regularly. With the membership came a personal trainer. I learned to use all the equipment and began to incorporate a healthier lifestyle. I felt great and used the excuse that it was a great way to delay my heart from failing. The truth was I was gaining the attention I lacked as a child, a bonus for me but a new addiction. Sometimes the kids would join me, which I thoroughly enjoyed, and once Ray came along. Just like skiing and snowmobiling my "new ways" were a bone of contention for him, yet I was intoxicated with my lifestyle. I didn't recognize it all lacked harmony.

Often I wondered why my husband wasn't attracted to me. I was pretty, smart, and had evolved into a confident, healthy woman. My baby fat was gone, my stomach was now flat, and I was proud to show it off with a belly piercing. Now, when I walked into a room, heads turned to acknowledge me, but not Ray's.

One weekend, a few friends were getting together for a party at a beach house. I had worn a peach bikini that accentuated every curve of my body. I was very proud of how I looked. We had gone swimming and when I came out of the water, I saw Ray point at another female on the beach while talking to my friend Matt.

As I approached, I heard him tell Matt, "Having a beautiful wife gets old and sometimes you need something new."

I continued to walk away without him noticing, hurt but after so many years of inattention, it no longer mattered. I was learning to love myself and make peace with myself and God. I wanted to surrender but was caught up in the multiple changes in my life providing me comfort.

I began to volunteer for a vacation plan called People and Places. I was a guide for people with disabilities. I found a new passion and I loved it! I felt energetic and more worthwhile than ever, and for the first time in a very long time I was happy!

I travelled the world and again asked Ray to participate. He once agreed and hated it!

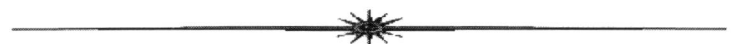

I had gained an exciting amount of confidence that surpassed any confidence I had known before. As a matter of fact, I probably became a little too cocky now as I used my new-found strength to begin to stand up to whomever I needed to, defending what I felt was right. You see at that time, I had a job that was quite enjoyable and was surrounded by great friends who I loved dearly but the supervisor was condescending and micromanaged us.

Although I loved my job, I reached a point where I would no longer turn my head and allow myself and my coworkers to be maltreated and disrespected. After living so many years of my own psychological abuse, seeds of hatred had been planted in my heart, and they were now projected onto my supervisor as the "straw that broke the camel's back." I had not felt that intensity of hatred toward anyone since my sister, Roberta.

Even after I left the job I dreamed my previous supervisor had been hit by a car. In the dream the police came to me as a suspect. I asked the officer how she died and he told me she died on impact. I responded, "No officer, if I had done it, it would've been a slow painful death." Subconsciously, I believe I had dreamed that because my marriage had become exactly that.

I landed on my feet as a nursing supervisor for a fairly new human services agency being trampled with state survey issues. I found a new purpose as a rescuer, a new avenue to hide my pain and I knew it.

Again I buried myself in a job that I loved and felt well-respected. I participated in many committees, created policies, and wanted my program to be equal or superior to others. I had a great team that was able to put systems in place in a very short period of time. I ran the agency's medical training program where I was proud to stand before both of my daughters as an educator when they became employed at the agency. It was cool to stand before them allowing them to see who I was in my professional life.

The agency ran like a well-oiled machine and the Director, Loren, allowed me to thrive. It was when she left the agency that confidence was again rocked. I had left my previous job over a difficult supervisor and had just regained my confidence. I had several supervisors after that and eventually grew tired of feeling helpless and stuck with each new layer. I decided that I would like to move up the corporate ladder and gain knowledge of the business itself. I made it a goal. When I expressed my goal to upper-level management I was told that I was good at what I did and should stay where I was. I felt I was being held back or put in a corner, again.

Now at 40-years-old, in 2004, I felt I had a career and marriage that were going nowhere and decided to improve myself professionally and spiritually. I needed to grow and began to explore my faith as well as expanding my intellectual knowledge. I learned about some free computer classes and began attending them every weekend. It was in class that I learned about their adult education classes, and the next thing I knew I was applying to be a student. Motivated by blind faith, I had no job plan; I had no plan at all, just felt compelled to do something. I was accepted and my life had new meaning!

In that classroom I met several adults from all aspects of life. It was a Christian program and we did a lot of improvisational speeches about ourselves, our lives, and our spiritual journey. I felt so safe in that setting and saw such passion among the other students. I learned about this new family in intimate ways that required no expectation from me. So many days I sat in awe listening, connecting to others like me.

We all shared in our desire to learn, shared in our goals, and gained strength through our experiences.

I was beginning to understand things slowly about myself. I was accepting of who I am and where I came from. I knew that I had good management skills that had grown out of my need to control my environment. I turned this weakness of needing to control into a positive by applying for a Bachelor's in Management program. Of course my self-discovery was still limited. I still needed to have people admire me. I still did not love myself or feel the power that

God from above loved me so divinely, I needed nothing more than to be myself, faults and all.

To this day I do not know what made me apply for a Bachelor's in Management instead of Nursing, but I know it was the best move I ever made and I believe God works in mysterious ways.

I knew I needed to move on personally, as well as professionally. I asked Ray for a divorce. It seemed to come out of nowhere to him and those around us. The past had been forgotten by all but me. I had raised my children and made one last ditch effort for him to become a bigger part of my life. I sat him down one day outlining what I needed from him: shared time, affection, mutual respect.

"There is nothing more I am willing to do for you," he responded that cold day in

November 2005.

It was clear our paths divided, our fate sealed. It was not until we parted that I realized he knew what I wanted all along. He wrote me letters clearly indicating things I believed he never knew. He knew I dreamed of having a real wedding with the white dress and my loved ones all around. Ours had been small, absent of our matriarchs, my Aunt Rita and his mother, both whom didn't accept our relationship. He knew I wanted the beautiful ring, the endless symbol of our love; my original had been stolen by his niece and I always felt it was Ray that should replace it as a gesture of renewal and commitment to us. He offered me this after I left. He knew I wanted to travel with him and offered to take me on a cruise. I cried for many days, recognizing all these years that he did know what I dreamed of yet held back. We could've had it all, we could've been married forever if only he had met me part of the way, acknowledged me. It was too little too late.

The kids were devastated, having thought the past had healed. I got hate mail and angry phone calls from them. I cried myself asleep many nights praying this would pass. I didn't understand! After all the years I had given up to provide for them how they could turn so quickly against me and hate me as they did. It was the most difficult time in my life!

Adam afforded me an opportunity for insight by writing a letter. It was painful for the kids to watch their father fall apart. I wrote him a letter in return explaining my story as politically correct as I could, choosing to remain neutral and loving toward their father. We had simply grown apart and made many mistakes along the way is what I told him.

Even Ray's friends tried to salvage our marriage. I was patient on Ray's behalf, struggling with knowing I had hurt him, guilty for his pain. The last paragraph in my marriage was in the presence of his friend Tom. I asked Ray three questions: "What is my favorite color, my favorite food, and my favorite song?" He was unable to answer any of them. After being together almost 26 years, not even trivial details mattered to him. His favorite color is blue, favorite food was steak, and favorite songs shared by Bob Dillon and Neil Young. He had always mattered to me.

When I left, I didn't look back to the pain and chose to give up the wonderful life I shared with my family in this chapter of my life. I was finally ready to move on. I believed I had "done my time," joking that marriage should be more like a car lease renewed routinely. I wish I was capable at the time to recognize "the car" I had chosen as a teenager could today be a classic, had I nurtured and loved it as it should've been.

Reflecting back, I can see where I became self-consumed. The power that I felt from creating my new life through work was invigorating. I became alive through work and going out, working out, skiing or snowboarding was like oxygen to me. I needed the thrill, glorification, and admiration I received. I was in control, demand. I was getting the attention that was deprived from my life.

Now, I do not need the excitement and I am not driven or concerned about what people think or need from me. I am learning to love myself and God. It's a slow process. Gradually, I am beginning to realize that my actions have caused pain and I have regrets. I am also too smart to let them consume me. I needed to leave Ray so he would love me, but I wish I would have done this in a different way. I would take the time to truly know myself before getting involved in another relationship and empower the relationships I have with my children before moving on. I would give everyone time to heal, including myself.

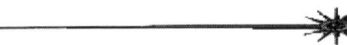

Reflection:

The years I was married to Ray were building blocks for the both of us. We both yearned to be loved, to be respected, and have importance in one another's lives. We were too young and stubborn to recognize that we both wanted the same things, and just couldn't reach one another to find it. Despite creating a home and our children, we grew apart. It is no fault on either of our part. We both experienced losses young in our lives and then fell into what soothed our emptiness.

Our marriage, like an ailing heart, did not have the tools of medical science to support a positive outcome. We had no medical options and no implantable devices to save us. As a result, we failed ourselves and one another. Fortunately, we were both able to let each other go allowing ourselves to love again in other relationships.

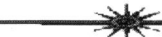

The best remedy for those who are afraid, lonely, or unhappy is to go outside, somewhere where they can be quiet, alone in the heavens, nature and God. Because only then does one feel that all is as it should be and that God wishes to see people happy, amidst the simple beauty of nature.

Ann Frank

POTHOLES

<u>A Triumphant Heart: Racing to the Finish Line:</u>

"I Promise Myself"

*To be so strong that nothing can
disturb my peace of mind.*

*To talk health, happiness, and prosperity
to every person I meet.*

*To make all my friends feel that there is
something worthwhile in them.*

*To look at the sunny side of everything
and make optimism come true.*

*To think only of the best, to work only for the best
and to expect only the best.*

*To be just as enthusiastic about the success of
others as I am about my own.*

*To forget the mistakes of the past and press on
to the greater achievements of the future.*

*To wear a cheerful expression at all times and
give a smile to every living creature I meet.*

*To give so much time to improving myself that
I have no time to criticize others.*

*To be too large for worry, too noble for anger,
too strong for fear, and too happy to
permit the presence of trouble.*

To think well of myself and to proclaim
this fact to the world,
not in loud words, but in great deeds.

To live in the faith that the whole world is on my side,
so long as I am true to the best that is in me.

Christian D. Larson

May 22, 2009

I was incredibly relieved that the first dose of medication went well–except for an excruciating headache that I wasn't sure what to pinpoint to. I thought maybe it was the result of an emotional let down from the build up to the procedure; pure anxiety was an emotion I hadn't dealt with in awhile. The doctors informed me that it may be the result of the enzymes and toxins produced as the medication destroyed my cells. I wondered if this is what it was like to receive chemotherapy.

Despite how I felt, I found out that Lauren was going to get her heart so I pleaded with the nurses to let me leave the floor for a few moments so that I could see her. I knew it was against their better judgment as I pleaded with them, but they seemed to understand my commitment to my family here. Like a child building parental trust, I gave them the room number I would be at, and had to take a note with me that had the unit phone number on it. I giggled like a mischievous child and headed on my way.

POTHOLES

Tearfully happy, I hugged Lauren and wished her well. It was if all of my emotions were thrown in one brief sitting. This was what we had all been waiting for, why I believed God had kept me here. Finally, we would all be on our way to recovery. I gave her the same advice Stephanie had given me about placing herself in God's hands. I hoped that she would find the same peace and faith in those words, and know He would carry her safely through.

As focused as I was on Lauren in our emotional moment, it was hard to ignore the ABC News cameras that were rolling behind us. I was all too familiar with their presence and knew Lauren would spend the next several hours completing intimate interviews with them. I excused myself in order to allow her sometime in the spotlight.

On the way back to my room I saw Lauren's family at the elevator. As I hugged them all we spotted a hawk circling at the windows. It was an interesting symbol.

When I returned to my room, I was flooded with exhaustion and pain. The side effects of the OKT3 were raging and the joints of my body throbbed with each beat of my new heart. I was proud of myself for enduring the first treatment as well as I did, and for the dedication to Lauren to forgo the pain long enough to support my "family." I allowed myself a few cleansing tears, wiped my slate clean for the day, and said my prayers for the night. I knew I could rest knowing God's plan would come to fruition and looked forward to the next day. I sent an e-mail to Julie to say hello and offer support before saying my prayers

+

May 23, 2009

I woke wondering how Lauren endured her surgery, but knew I would get no information unless I walked over to the unit to see her family. There, I saw her name on the patient care board, and was able to peek in on her through the glass walls. She slept peacefully as her family gathered around her donned in the hospital gowns, gloves, and masks required after surgery. We shared joyful glances and I continued on my way.

As I walked back to my room I reminisced about the stories we had all shared and recalled Jackie's seemingly tireless efforts to ensure Lauren's needs were met. Despite working a full-time job, she never missed an opportunity to prepare a healthy, home cooked meal for her only daughter, yet would frequently fall asleep at the bedside after providing care to her. Lauren felt confused as to why her mom just didn't stay home, but I understood as a mother.

Jackie's desire was to encourage Lauren to eat and remain strong despite her grueling nausea. I ate out of necessity, but Lauren was often too tired or weak. I think it frightened us all watching her grow weaker by the day. I couldn't imagine what it must've been like for Jackie, watching helplessly. I knew too well that level of powerlessness with my own genetic blueprint. I hoped I could be that dedicated for my own children's future.

Jackie would speak lovingly about her frustration with those little things that frustrated "us" patients, and how they would bicker over Lauren's need to control the environment. This I understood, oh too well!

"Sometimes I would be exhausted after working all day, cooking for Lauren, and then staying at the hospital before returning home to my husband. Lauren would want me to wash her hair or bathe her and sometimes I just didn't have the energy. When Lauren would complain, I wanted to pull her hair, but just made faces behind her back," she would joke.

"One time I fell asleep in the recliner and Lauren got mad at me," Jackie laughed.

"Ma, you are here to visit me. Go home if you are tired," Lauren would tell her.

Lauren didn't understand why her mother just didn't stay home, but I understood. Not only did I understand, but I knew that someday I may be standing next to Erin or Adam with that same level of devotion.

"One time I made the mistake of making a mess with popcorn and Lauren was furious. Yeah! I understand that control thing!" Jackie laughed.

Lauren was in the hospital almost four months and her mom repeated the ritual day after day: work, preparing dinner, assisting Lauren and preparing her for bed, then heading home, praying to arrive safely in order to prepare dinner for her husband, and prepare for another day.

By the time I arrived back to my room, my spirits were lifted and I embraced my next dose of OKT3. Following the dose I experienced a cocktail of flu-like symptoms, nausea, stomach distress, and headaches making it a very busy night in and out of the bathroom.

With little time to prepare my heart for quick jaunts to the bathroom, I found myself getting light-headed and needing to duck my head between my knees to keep from passing out. Once I'd fall back into bed the heart would still be racing because of the adrenaline, and it would take a very long time to relax. With the culmination of medications, side effects, fatigue, and possibly dehydration, I wondered how much more my body could endure.

Throughout most of the next day, I did very little. Many people suggested I treat myself to a retreat day and I thought, *that's a great idea!* I put my relaxation music on and felt so tired and weak I couldn't muster up enough energy to change the channel. I only rolled out of bed when necessary, and struggled when dialing the phone to order food. When I regained some strength, I trudged over to my couch to lay on it in the sun taking in its warmth. I treated myself to a day without expectation.

Overall, the residual from the medicine was unbearable. It was the worst I had felt since I was admitted to the hospital with my failing, broken heart. None of the medication offered relieved the excruciating pain in my joints; radiating in every vertebra in my neck, down my back, and into my lower legs. I would sit for hours massaging whatever I could reach, trying to dissipate the inflammation. As the day drew to a close I recognized one more dose was behind me. I planned on a good night's rest and a much better tomorrow!

I hadn't heard from Dr. Ken's family, but Lauren's mom Jackie stopped in. She brought me some cookies, which was truly comforting since I hadn't left my room for a while. I so much appreciated her company and the update on Lauren. They were elated with her progress, and once again, I was invited to share in their joy.

It was then I recognized the wealth that God had blessed me with. To this point, I had been fortunate enough to share intimately in the lives of six families' success stories, filled with tears of fear, disappointment, laughter, and joy. It was incomprehensible to me to feel so overwhelmingly supported by those who were going through so much themselves. I had gained so much from knowing them; I felt God couldn't have been any more generous. I sat down to blog and e-mail Julie.

May 24, 2009

Today was my daughter Amanda's twenty-fifth birthday and despite being in the hospital, I was happy to be alive for this milestone. I was also happy to say, as Geoff so eloquently put it, "Montezuma's Revenge" seems to have "exited" quietly. I started the day a little dehydrated, my electrolytes seemed off, I was fairly lethargic, had quite the headache, and such a painfully stiff neck and back. I'd had Tylenol most of the day and pushed fluids on top of adding the potassium and magnesium doses. Of course with all the steroids, my blood sugars were a little higher which added to my sluggishness, and my cheeks were flushed.

I pushed myself to shower, then wrapped myself in a flannel bed sheet and sat in my recliner to do my morning buffing and puffing. I probably looked like Cleopatra when the nurses and aides came in for their morning routine! The rest of the day was fairly painless and non-productive.

Anna, one of the nurses, offered to give me my next dose of medication earlier than usual because my sleep cycle had been confused, somewhat like a baby. I was sleeping off the Benadryl during the day and up in pain all night. I found it amusing and giggled at how nervous each nurse became when administering the OKT3 for the first time. Sometimes I felt helpful explaining to the nurses how to administer it because it required a special I.V. filter. Today's dose went well, and Anna appeared relieved. I lay in bed for almost four hours napping on and off deciding I liked Benadryl!

The aches and pains again returned but were less in intensity. I felt well enough to take a walk trying to tire myself and burn off some glucose from the cookies I snacked on after dinner! It also gave me an excuse to peek in on Lauren.

As I passed, she was awake! I said hello through the door and marveled at her pink cheeks and brilliant blue sparkling eyes. When she smiled at me, her smile lit up the room. I was so happy to be here to see her on this side of her journey.

Awhile later, I got a wonderful visit from Surrinder. We shared a cup of tea. Dr. Ken was having a better day and I hoped both of us would be up to a visit the next day. Some nurses from the other floors also came to visit and my final visitor for the day was my doctor.

He told me my most recent biopsy actually looked good. The heart was not showing signs of rejection only healing now! I thought, *Yay! May I repeat, Yay! Again, Yay!* He continued to say that my cell counts were also significantly reducing and things seemed to be heading in the right direction. They planned to continue this med for seven days, repeat the biopsy and MRI then determine the course of action from there. I was ecstatic and went to sleep knowing I would be on my way soon. I was thankful for every moment, every opportunity, and every life lesson!

May 25, 2009

I woke during the night in pain greater than I had ever imagined. I began to explore a reason for the side effects and ways to alleviate my discomfort to no avail. I called the nurse and tried a few different pain medications, including something for anxiety. I even tried elevating my still throbbing legs on the bedside table. I was now hyper, wide-awake, and in a ridiculous position in bed. I laughed at my conundrum and began to think about what could be causing such untouchable discomfort! I thought maybe my liver was overwhelmed from all of the medication or something was toxic! In the morning, my blood level came back high, so I thought, perhaps it was the problem.

When Surrinder dropped by that morning, the pain and fatigue was apparent. She began to massage my back and I melted under her warm, gentle hands. It felt great to be pampered. I hadn't had a backrub since I was in the unit. After our visit, I decided I would go for a walk myself. I went to see Phil but his door was closed, and Lauren was sleeping. I walked a little more then decided to check in and visit Dr. Ken. We joked about experiences, our "potholes," deciding it was best to jump them!

I walked back toward Phil's room and the nurse asked if I was Linda. She said he tried to walk to my room today but it was too far for him. With that news, I turned around and I visited him. I was amazed at his progress! He was exuberant! He said he felt great and was thrilled I stopped by to visit. He planned to visit my room tomorrow.

Lauren was still asleep so I waved as I passed and headed back to my room. I missed the sunset, but there was the most beautiful complete rainbow across the entire sky that seemed to last forever. I just sat awestruck thinking, *what a completely, wonderful, miraculous, world it is!*

Before I fell asleep, my nurse gave me another backrub and at that very moment I was calm, relaxed, and almost pain free. That was miraculous too!

May 26, 2009

It was a beautiful and sunny day in Boston. I thought about sneaking outside briefly, but it had been really hard to get up and moving after another painful night. My knees and legs were again throbbing, and were inflamed and hot to the touch. I was incredibly uncomfortable. The doctors said it was Fibromyalgia from the medicine and should resolve once the treatments were done. I endured it as long as I could during the night but gave in to the pain after propping my hips up on the bedside table again, this time on a pillow, with no relief. I'm sure I looked ridiculous, but just couldn't get comfortable!

I literally hobbled like "Estelle Geddy" to the nurses' station and graciously accepted back-to-back doses of Dilaudid that barely took the edge off. My mentality had become to sleep when I could as I did in my child-rearing days.

The salvation of my morning was a wonderfully hot shower. I flung my exhausted body over the shower chair where I remained motionless as the heat engulfed my aches. By the time I got out and dressed, I felt whole again and it was time for the usual medication routine and a nap.

To my delight, Phil popped in around 3 p.m. He had indeed met his goal of being able to walk far enough to see me! By 4 p.m. I was able to get up and moving, finally. I stopped by to visit Dr. Ken and did a "wave by" to Lauren. Today is an absolutely wonderful day. All of my friends are doing great including the ones who have headed home. I still hadn't heard from Julie but I decided I'd ask Kristyn for assistance the next day.

I was cautiously optimistic about the possibility of a peaceful night's sleep or another shower, even if I had to sleep in there!

May 27, 2009

I actually slept three hours and was thrilled to wake late; at almost 4 a.m. I rested until a reasonable hour to start my day. There was a little glitch with the OKT3 and they were unable to draw the full dose up due to not having enough supply. I was all woozy on my Benedryl cocktail. *How can a hospital not have enough medication?* I thought.

They opted to give me a "short dose" for the day and tomorrow would be the last. I wondered if a "short dose" would mean less pain.

I napped it all off very willingly and crawled out of bed around 4 p.m. ABC News and several other visitors were in. Phil even walked by, but he wanted nothing to do with the video cameras! I had noticed that fear of television cameras had been an epidemic here, considering the hospital was hosting a documentary.

I felt well enough to leave the floor, and headed to the Family Center. I knew from past experience, that cookies were delivered in the afternoon. I chose chocolate chip ones to take to Phil and Lauren. We visited briefly and I was off! I spent some time reading and relaxing, but it is difficult to remain focused. The doctors were very pleased with how well I was tolerating it all and have me cautiously optimistic about discharge on Friday. Monica, the pharmacist, refers to me as a "superstar" because of all I have endured: I guess I am! I had more tests scheduled, so I asked my friends and family to: "Call in their Angels for me."

May 28, 2009

I have spent a lot of time reflecting over some of the sillier moments that I have been experiencing lately, the most prevalent is the hand tremor. It made simple tasks monumental and hand-eye coordination was long gone.

My favorite example was putting on my eye makeup, which would have me laughing hysterically at myself. I would end up looking like a deranged "Betty Boop!" Between the bad makeup and the facial swelling we had a striking resemblance. With my new look, Chris began calling me "Nanook!"

The medications now created expansive mood swings and I confided in Chris that I'd developed a short fuse for basic stupidity. An aide came in after I had come back from a long walk to alleviate some of the anxiety and wanted to check my vitals. I graciously got into my recliner and put my feet up to accommodate her. At that point my heart was still racing because I failed to cool down from my walk. She stood across the room at bedside looking at me and said, "Can you come over here? I don't feel like moving the blood pressure cuff."

    I felt a rush of hot blood surge through my veins and to the tips of my ears in disbelief at what I had heard: steroid rage! I know it was a silly thing but I was incredibly edgy. I took a deep breath knowing this emotion was new to me, but my lips started to hiss like hot bacon. "You certainly could've moved the cuff for me Missy!" I said. Afterward I prayed that I could control myself over such trivial things in the future. It was going to be a rough ride.

    I threatened to kill Chris on the phone when he told me he wanted to mow the perennial ground cover flower beds alongside the house and plant grass. I wondered who was the crazy one, me or him, and why anyone would want to set me off like that! I needed another prayer!

    Ordering food now felt like a "Deal a meal" adventure. I don't think there was anyway to order where the meal could turn out right. It was either a mystery meal or a cruel trick. I would order chicken pasta broccoli and get spaghetti! I thought it was a conspiracy and prayed repeatedly my manners would stay in check.

    I was now able to lay flat on my back in bed for the first time stretching out my abdomen. I was amused at myself at the things I had taken for granted. I tried sleeping on my side, but the pressure on the healing chest bones made it unbearable. I was ready for my last dose of OKT3 and wondered how much better I will feel once the toxins worked their way out of my body. I imagined the possibilities!

My friends Phil and Dr. Ken were pending being discharged along with me on Friday and my friend Lauren was right behind us! It seemed a beautiful end to this saga; a great ending, but a beautiful beginning for the entire group that endured this together.

May 29, 2009

Tick-Tock, the clock kept marching on. I was thrilled to find out I was on the biopsy schedule for 9 a.m., so I was up, showered, and in my "hospital clothes" ready to go. I planned ahead knowing I would miss breakfast, and walked to the Family Center prior to stash a juice and muffin for when I returned.

The procedure went well and I was back to the floor in less than thirty minutes. The nurse was shocked to see me. To pass time I took a wonderful long walk, did some stairs, and watched a movie. I was fortunate to run into a few folks along the way.

Phil was doing awesome and announced he was going to get married. He proposed to his girlfriend and was on "Cloud Nine!" It seemed to be a nice story. He told me they had broken up out of anger when he learned he was ill. He gave her no explanation. When she found out what had occurred, she committed herself to being a part of his journey. Emotions ran high for the two of them and I wondered if the timing was good to make such a serious decision.

I learned later that his discharge to home had been delayed because of concerns with his blood pressure and swelling in his feet. I reminded him that it was better to be cautious at this time. Of course, he was not happy. I believe though, that his family was in agreement with the doctors and grateful for their decision.

Dr. Ken was in the hall walking for the first time, another triumph! I think I was so delighted; I skipped back to my room. I planned to stop back later to say our goodbyes.

For that moment, I cautiously packed and organized to go home, but remained in a self-protect mode. Chris and his dad were coming in to prepare potentially for my return home. I was excited about saying goodbye to the ABC news team again and the Brigham team hopefully this time for real. It was a great place to stay, but I didn't want to live there anymore!

May 30, 2009

Today would be my discharge day, pending all going well. It was a gut-wrenching wait for the biopsy results. I was afraid to get my hopes up, fearing disappointment again. The ABC News folks were there again, and Valery was doing the exit interviews. We did lots of walking around the floors, and saying goodbyes. Lauren and I exchanged hugs and signatures on our "heart" pillows given to cardiac patients after surgery. The pillows were used by the surgeons to outline the procedure they completed on you. Ours were blank because we had entirely new hearts. Dr. Couper, my surgeon, signed mine, "Do Great Things," and notified us the biopsy was clean! You cannot imagine my relief! I fell happily backward onto my bed!

Kristyn my Social Worker and Katherine the Chaplain came in while I was doing a "happy dance." A few nurses slid a note under the door because they didn't want anything to do with the news team. My father-in-law wanted nothing to do with the cameras either and told them, "I was getting a lot of attention for someone who had their appendix out!" It was pretty funny. We waited till 2:30 p.m. before they actually let me go. By then, I took my own telemetry off and I.V. out. We really didn't want to get caught in the rush hour on a Friday night in Boston traffic; especially during Red Sox season and on Memorial Day weekend. This year, we really had something to celebrate.

I was trying valiantly to leave graciously, and not melt down in front of everyone. Until then, most of my tears had been hidden. When it was time to leave, I got into the wheelchair and told Valery, "I am trying so hard not to cry." She looked at me endearingly and said, "Linda, after all you have been through, it is alright to cry." Perhaps I just needed permission, for the tears began to flow freely. This time, they were tears of joy. I forgot to ask about Julie but vowed I would.

The ride was not bad, about 6.5 hours, but with all the joint pain from the meds, I was somewhat uncomfortable. We got home a little after 10 p.m. I walked into my home and sighed with relief. I said to Chris, "I had forgotten how much I love it here." I was greeted happily from the boys, and was happy to be where I belonged: home with my family; who could ask for anything more? Looking at it from his point of view, I agree with my friend Kenny, "There's no place like home!"

Reflection:

When Dr. Couper gave me my pillow, he thought for quite a while before he wrote, "Do great things." While leaving the hospital I wondered what God had in mind for me. What could I do that would be so profound, deserving this second chance at life? Each day I woke appreciating this beautiful world and recounting my blessings. I looked at local events, volunteer work, and multiple organizations that I could feel passionate about being a part of. It was stressful and pressured. I realized that just as I had watched Dr. Couper take the time to develop his thoughts, I too was entitled to the same.

I realized I needed to surrender it to God and when He was ready; I would be shown the way. I discovered that I can do great things everyday by simply treating everyone well, inspiring others, and teaching from my experiences. I recalled the term "Pay it Forward," from so long ago and am committed to doing things for others every single day including treating them with respect, and giving of myself. Whether it is a shoulder to cry on, an ear to listen, or a voice of reason, it doesn't have to be monumental. I recalled a simple quote by Mother Theresa, "We can do no great things, only small things with great love." This is what I aspire to do for now, and I'll take it!

My great hope is to laugh as much as I cry; to get my work done and try to love somebody and have the courage to accept love in return.

Maya Angelou

Chapter 14

A Second Chance at Life

When a heart fails and can no longer be managed through medication, a transplant may be the next option. Depending on the history and progression of the heart's failure, each person's path can be very different. The wait can be painstakingly short or long depending upon the outlook. Every aspect of one's life becomes affected, scrutinized very closely.

The transplant list is layered based on medical acuity and hospitalization status. In the best possible scenario, intravenous medication can promote a sense of well-being while waiting for a new organ. There is no standard progression, nothing predictable; we are all unique in our journey.

I was lucky. My heart failed slowly which allowed me plenty of time to adjust and for my body to accommodate to its changes. I functioned well until just a few months before I was hospitalized for the final steps. Up until then, I worked and lived a productive life. I was blessed.

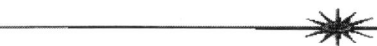

I am a hopeless romantic. I don't know why, as love has failed me on so many levels; or perhaps I have failed it. To be honest, I am afraid to love fully. Most everything I have loved, or was supposed to be able to count on in my life had somehow failed. Some was through no fault of my own. I had no control over the loss of my parents, my sister, or even my first spouse. I didn't realize that my love for life and family had actually been a catalyst in our eventual break up. I have grown a great deal since then and hope that my understanding of the many loves in our lives will find a way to benefit others as well.

I am not alone in my wants and desires. Everybody wants happiness and longs for love. I had hopes, dreams, and ambitions and now I realize new dreams. In Buddhism, it is said that each person is born with so many breaths. After that, they pass into the afterlife. As I became older this became true for me: only it was so many beats. It was time to let go and make my life magical.

In theory, Ray and I had it all, three beautiful children who were almost grown, a house near the lake, steady jobs, and our health but my heart knew the truth. There was too much betrayal. Part of me wanted to stay. In theory our lives should be renewed. It should've been enough, yet I wanted more.

How did I get so caught up in the fairytale-life with so little love? Where did I lose my insight with God? Was I that desperate? It took me years to realize how good I was at the appearance of having it all together. Inside, it was all a lie.

I was that weak female with low self-esteem that wanted nothing more than to be loved at any cost. In fact, so much so that I believe my heart could have bled tears. I knew what was right but was willing to give up my dreams for love and for the feeling of being safe and secure. This was the mantra I realized to be most significant to me later in life. What was very fortunate for me was that somehow all of the situations that could've gone terribly bad ended up finding their way to a brighter side.

I realized that I escaped into skiing, snowmobiling, and happy hours that only lead nowhere. The excitement was only temporary. I loved the rush of snowmobiling and skiing that allowed for the connection to nature. I could gather my thoughts there, but my thoughts continued to push me forward. I needed a challenge that sports could not provide. I went back to school where all my dreams could come true.

Going back to school signified a new beginning for me, not simply a new chapter, but a new book entirely. I wasn't sure where I was headed or what I wanted to do, maybe I was looking for another escape from home.

When I first noticed Chris, my impression of him was that his appearance resembled his life; in order, unlike mine. He was the only student not dressed casually; perhaps that's why I noticed him in particular. I was cynical, thinking that he must be really vain dressing that way appearing to maintain positional power above the rest of us. A few short weeks into our studies, we were asked to give an impromptu speech which involved taking a personal item in our possession and talking about it for a few minutes. It was a spur of the moment, on the spot assignment.

I happened to have a gold earring in my purse from my sister Patti. I had lost one, but carried the other believing that metal held her memory. My story involved losing that earring a few years prior and how I came to find it outside my home while I was hosing dirt from my shoes. I never questioned how it got there, just accepted it as a gift from heaven.

Chris pulled a worry stone out of his pocket given to him by his young son Evan. He spoke about this endearingly and carried it everywhere he went. I noticed the kindliness in his green eyes; and as he spoke, they twinkled beneath his tinted glasses.

I did not intend to meet someone at school. I wanted to empower myself, heal, and move on, but Chris disarmed me. He was engaging and provided me with warmth that I desired. He listened intently when I talked and looked me in the eyes. When I talked he stopped whatever he was doing to offer his undivided attention to me, and I liked the feeling of importance. As the weeks progressed, speeches included our goals, spiritual journey, and what we held dear to us. The classroom grew intimate and I found myself sharing things about myself without reservation. I didn't have to pretend to be happy and was allowed to be human. The environment was safe and non-threatening.

I learned that Chris's goal was to become a hospital administrator and that he had recently quit smoking. He didn't want his boys to learn from this example and even though he had smoked for 20 years, he loved his boys, Grant and Evan, enough for the sacrifice! I was impressed that he admitted to making bad decisions and righting them again.

Sometimes when he talked there was a sharp, tense edge about him which confused me. He was definitely someone I could welcome in my life after living through a bad marriage, but I was afraid he may have a temper.

One day Chris approached me and out of the blue asked me, "What makes women so suspicious and judgmental?"

I replied, "Men they can't trust."

He confided in me that he was going through a difficult divorce of a failed second marriage. His soon to be ex-wife had a history of dating married men and this had been a hurdle for trust in their marriage. I reflected on my own life including failed marriages, infidelity, and lack of trust. I hugged him and told him to hang in there.

A few weeks later, the seat next to me in class became available and Chris moved from his seat in the right front row next to mine. I learned that he was going to be celebrating his 40th birthday and I associated the number with a milestone in any life and in the Bible, I gave him *The Purpose Driven Life,* by Rick Warren, a gift I had received for my 40th birthday. Often when we would talk I would playfully suggest that because I was older, I was wiser.

There was a day this mentality was halted with his well-thought response: "You do realize that we are only nine months apart? Did you ever think I was conceived to be with you?" he continued. "Do you think maybe there was a purpose that we met in a period of time when we both were forty?" he asked me.

I didn't know how to respond to his positive attention and perceived spiritual depth and insight.

A few nights after school, the group went out together. We learned more about one another through casual conversation in a more relaxed environment. I still found Chris to be intense, but charming and attentive. I liked that.

He learned quickly what my favorite things were. Getting together as a couple at this point was not at all my intention.

One Friday night while I was heading home my cell phone rang. It was Chris asking if I wanted to stop by to watch the hockey game. I was curious about him and for whatever reason headed there. His boys, Grant who was 8-years-old and Evan who was 11-years-old, were home so it was safe. We ended up having a snowball fight with them. We all ganged up on Chris using garbage cans lids as shields and ran around the neighboring yards. Chris looked at me in the light of the streetlights and said, "You're just a big kid!"

He was right. For years I had suppressed the mischievous, fun-loving little girl in me and I took this opportunity to let her out. I felt comfortable doing so in his presence. I recalled a quote by an unknown author, "It's never too late to have a happy childhood, but the second one is up to you and no one else." I was ready to take a chance.

The next day, Chris called to talk about whether I thought we might be ready for a relationship or not. It took me by surprise. He wanted to make it clear that he had children and they would be a part of our lives and he was not interested in bringing women in and out of their lives. I admired him for that.

I enjoyed his company and admired how well he managed a home, a job, school, and children on his own. His house was tidy, tastefully decorated, and welcoming. I was quite impressed with a man that could do it all himself and didn't require me to rescue him. Looking back, I find he was like my Uncle Lee, and maybe I was like my mom just looking for the perfect man to take care of me. I give his mother Karen a great deal of credit for supporting him through it all. She offered Chris and the boys' stability when things fell apart. She took on a parental role with the kids and made sure nothing fell through the cracks. She was always there.

I learned that Chris' first wife left when the boys were just eighteen months and 3- years-old. She simply wasn't prepared to be a mother and fell into the graces of another man. I tried not to place judgment, but from a woman's point of view it was unfathomable: they were babies. For me it was incomprehensible.

I wasn't naive, I recognized there were two sides to this story, just like my marriage, and I knew by then how powerful new love could be. What I had difficulty with understanding was whether new love was more powerful than the love of your children. I can't judge, I left Ray; I walked away and yes my kids were adults, but was it the same?

I fell in love with Chris almost immediately, almost becoming addicted. I loved his soothing and gentle voice. He looked at me lovingly, something I hadn't seen in Ray's eyes for so long. I loved watching him iron his clothes, perfectly pressing in the pleats. I loved the way he did laundry, the way he cooked. Everything he did was done with passion and patience. I believed God had placed his hand in my destiny.

There were no secrets between us; we started the relationship with our darkest most intimate details on the table, including our fears. I had no fear with Chris and felt in him I had everything I could possibly ask for. He learned of my heart condition and like most others assumed it wouldn't happen for many years. It was brutally, beautifully honest.

There wasn't a time we were together he didn't hold my hand, open a door, or kiss me good night. As cliché as it was, he seemed to complete me. Our lives together were simple with few worries. He took care of me and expected little in return. We were alike in our methodical ways yet complimented one another in our sense of urgency. I had a fear of not getting things done and he took his time. He was the only person I ever knew who was able to help me see the joy in simply enjoying the moment.

On our first date I told him my favorite song was, "Bohemian Rhapsody," by Queen. The next day, he handed me a gift. Guess what it was? To date, if that song comes on the radio, he instinctively calls me or turns it up. He learned my favorite color is white, and I love snowmen because they are always so happy. The first Christmas we dated, he bought me a gold snowman necklace; simple things, but important to me.

He asked me to come live with him much sooner than I could've expected. I accepted. It wasn't long after when one night he simply sat up, resting on his heels and asked me to marry him. It was the epitome of a whirlwind relationship and I sunk like the *Titanic!* I loved him so purely and deeply, more than I could comprehend. He allowed for stability and stirred up my childhood desires. He wanted me, desired me, and loved me. In his proposal, he promised a big, white wedding. I was thrilled to say, "Yes, Yes, Yes!" My childhood dream came true in the summer of 2007. It was a day that I will treasure for a lifetime. I felt like a princess walking through the flower gardens of Niagara Falls in my own beautiful white dress. For that one day, Cinderella had found her handsome prince.

My hair was pulled up in tendrils that filled my rhinestone tiara and I wore a necklace and earrings I'd borrowed from Amanda that glimmered like diamonds. My "Maid of Honor," my friend Melissa, was a stanchion of support and made sure everything went perfectly. All of our kids and grandkids, brothers, and sisters were a part of the ceremony. The girls wore peridot gowns and the men wore black tuxes. It was a fall wedding, so the earth tones set a very warm tone for flowers, table cloths and the cake. I couldn't have been any happier, or anymore complete.

Chris was trembling. Our two lives and our families were now woven into one.

Until that day, however, lurking inside my head was a nagging thought. Had I healed enough or was I repeating the same pattern my mother did when she married my Uncle Lee? When I saw him that day waiting my question was answered.

Reality quickly set in after the wedding. Chris was the caring father I had never known. I admired how he took full responsibility for the welfare of the children. I did not agree with all his methods, but admired his determination.

I was now in the trenches of being the step-parent and gained a new respect for Carla, who had been my step-mother for those nine years. Chris' children seemed as determined to make sure they didn't leave room in their life for me as I did with Carla. I realized her sacrifices and understood the difficulty in raising children who cautiously welcomed you, if they welcomed you at all. At the time I came into their lives, these guys had established personalities, and their male rituals were the entombed, similar to how I was with Carla. They loved television, video games, and fast food and I felt I'd stepped back into the days when I took care of Perry. They believed my job as the woman of the house was to cook, clean, and take care of them. We all had a rude awakening and God was blessing me with an opportunity to see it through this time!

Chris, who eagerly wanted a happy life together as a family with raising the children, was quickly disillusioned, especially as my health began to fail. My heart was wearing out as quickly as my dreams.

With my new heart came new realities. I know now that there should be three in a marriage. The couple themselves and God to keep them together. I know that life is not perfect but everyday life can be fulfilling. I appreciate Chris for all that he has given of himself to help me to heal. He and his family were supportive of me when I went to Boston. I had so much support from my family, my children, all of my friends, and so many others. When I returned home, I did not simply have a new heart, but a new vision. The vision was to recreate my life and empower others to do the same.

Mine is not a perfect life nor is it a perfect marriage. If it were I'd have no lessons left to learn. Chris and I are learning more and more about one another everyday, hopefully continuing to grow together instead of apart. The glue of our relationship to this point has been God's presence in our lives.

Reflection:

There is no right, wrong, or better way of doing things. It is not our right to judge others. That is reserved for God. The paths we choose and the lessons we learn are all uniquely our own. We hope that through our experiences we can help others, save them from pain, provide them comfort, or catch them when they fall. I have often failed; failed to see myself from the perspective of others, failed to look within myself for understanding, and failed to practice the lessons I have learned. I understand I have a long way to go to heal as I did when I was in the hospital waiting for my heart. I am happy to explore myself from a different point of view on the wings of my second chance.

Although I joke with Chris about visual decline that comes with the age of forty, simple magnifying glasses can assist you to see the world outside. No magnifying glass known to man can help you though with patterns of the heart. It is the ability to look within that becomes our most significant accomplishment.

Here I was once again trying to go on with my life, reflecting how it had come "full circle." Nothing in life should have greater value than your faith. When your faith is strong, your ability to love, trust, and be patient becomes instinctively natural. This time God would be at the forefront of my life. He is truly my savior. I now believe that "The Fairytale" was created for the purpose of finding someone to share my life with. All princesses overcame obstacles before the "Happily Ever After," and I am no different.

God is a given in our lives. He was there in my weakest moments, the one I prayed to when I was brought to my knees, the one who sent me peaceful and beautiful messages to get me through.

Happiness lies for those who cry, those who hurt, those who have searched, and those who have tried for only they can appreciate the importance of people who have touched their lives.

Unknown

When all is said and done:

Many cultures believe that the heart is the key to wellness, as do I. I read once that the heart possesses its own intelligence and the ability to house the very emotions that affect our day-to-day lives. Vitality, productivity, and relationships are keys of the heart. It is a scientific fact that the heart's electromagnetic field is 60-times stronger than the brain's and it can impact every cell in your body

There is no question that the state of our heart impacts our overall well-being: both when in love and in pain. When your heart is healthy, strong and open, your body follows.

I was able to connect a few more times via e-mail with Julie and we continued to share our journeys the encompassing months. She would often comment on my blog about how happy she was that I had my life back. Usually, I would send her a separate more personal correspondence to simply "be available" to her. Although she wasn't part of my "transplant family," she became a part of me. I felt connected to her.

Julie represented the part of transplant surgery that no one likes to talk about: the patient that was unable to be saved, the reason we all need to donate organs. This young mother passed away shortly after I was discharged from the hospital. She died at home with her family and very peaceful...just like my mother.

POTHOLES

Afterthoughts:

To realize
The value of a sister/brother

Ask someone
Who doesn't have one.

To realize
The value of ten years:
Ask a newly
Divorced couple.

To realize
The value of four years:
Ask a graduate.

To realize
The value of one year:
Ask a student who
Has failed a final exam.

To realize
The value of nine months:
Ask a mother who gave birth to a stillborn.

To realize
The value of one month:
Ask a mother
Who has given birth to
A premature baby.

When All is Said and Done

To realize
The value of one week:
Ask an editor of a weekly newspaper.

To realize
The value of one minute:
Ask a person
Who has missed the train, bus or plane.

To realize
The value of one-second:
Ask a person
Who has survived an accident.

Time waits for no one.
Treasure every moment you have.

You will treasure it even more when
You can share it with someone special.

To realize the value of a friend or family member:
LOSE ONE.

-unknown

Pot holes can be repaired but the road is forever changed.

12674935R00201

Made in the USA
Charleston, SC
19 May 2012